Chicken Soup for the Soul®

Say Goodbye to Stress

Chicken Soup for the Soul: Say Goodbye to Stress
Manage Your Problems, Big and Small, Every Day
by Dr. Jeff Brown with Liz Neporent

Published by Chicken Soup for the Soul Health, an imprint of Chicken Soup for the Soul Publishing,
LLC www.chickensoup.com
Copyright © 2012 by Chicken Soup for the Soul Publishing, LLC. All Rights Reserved.

Front cover and interior photo courtesy of iStockphoto.com/imagedepotpro.
Back cover photo of Dr. Jeff Brown © Eric Laurits.

Cover and Interior Design & Layout by Pneuma Books, LLC
For more info on Pneuma Books, visit www.pneumabooks.com

Distributed to the booktrade by Simon & Schuster. SAN: 200-2442

Publisher's Cataloging-In-Publication Data
(Prepared by The Donohue Group, Inc.)

Brown, Jeff (Jeffrey Lowell), 1969-

Chicken soup for the soul : say goodbye to stress : manage your problems, big and small, every day
/ by Jeff Brown with Liz Neporent.

p. ; cm.

Summary: A collection of stories on the topic of reducing and managing stress, accompanied by
medical advice.

ISBN: 978-1-935096-88-7

1. Stress management--Popular works. 2. Stress management--Anecdotes. I. Neporent, Liz. II. Title.
III. Title: Say goodbye to stress

PN6071.S73 B76 2012
810.2/02/356/1   2012931533

PRINTED IN THE UNITED STATES OF AMERICA
on acid∞free paper

21 20 19 18 17 16 15 14 13 12   01 02 03 04 05 06 07 08 09 10

Chicken Soup for the Soul.

Say Goodbye to Stress

Manage Your Problems, Big and Small, Every Day

by **DR. JEFF BROWN** of
HARVARD MEDICAL SCHOOL
with **LIZ NEPORENT**

Chicken Soup for the Soul Publishing, LLC
Cos Cob, CT

Chicken Soup for the Soul®

www.chickensoup.com

Contents

Chapter 3

～ **Killer Jobs — Stress and the Workplace** ～

Chapter 4

～ **Home Is Where the Heat Is** ～

Chapter 5

～ **Preventing Monetary Meltdown** ～

Chapter 6

～ **Emotions and Thoughts** ～

Chapter 7
〜 **Mind Your Stress** 〜

Chapter 8
〜 **De-stress Your Lifestyle** 〜

Introduction

O rganizational psychologist Cary Cooper, a leading authority on workplace stress, once noted that stress is the "black plague" of our times. He believes that stress is the main source of, or the trigger for, disease in the 21st century developed world. It's hard to argue with Cooper when the link between stress and just about every major disease or illness is so well established.

Stress is a global epidemic. The most recent National Health Interview Survey reported that more than 75 percent of people feel stressed out during any given two-week time frame, with about half the population admitting to experiencing frequent moderate-to-high levels of stress during that time. Workers' compensation claims related to stress and mental health have gone through the roof in the last thirty years; some states report a 700 percent rise in claims even as other claim categories have remained flat or declined.

And as Cooper points out, all this negative emotion is taking a heavy toll. Financially speaking, it costs American companies nearly $300 billion a year to address the claims, lost productivity and missed days of work of their stressed-out workforce. Medically speaking, the American Medical Association reports that at least 60 percent of all illness can trace its roots back to the negative effects of stress; a 20-year study conducted by the University of London concluded that unmanaged reactions to stress were a more dangerous risk factor for cancer and heart disease than either cigarette smoking or high cholesterol foods. And personally speaking, it's impossible to put a price tag on just how deeply stress ravages individuals, families and relationships.

We wrote this book to show you that you are not alone in feeling overwhelmed and undone by life—and also to show you that stress isn't a foregone conclusion. As the stories in this book and the scientific information we've provided illustrate, there are some concrete and proactive steps you can take to reduce the stress you feel and the way stress affects you. Most of the time you can't change the world around you, but we think it's important for you to know that you can change your reaction to it.

So read on to see how regular folks like you and me have invented some ingenious workarounds to the stress in their lives. Then read the explanations of why these often simple strategies can work for you too. I think the power of storytelling backed up with well-established medical facts can help you manage the stress in your life no matter what source it comes from.

~ Jeff Brown, Psy.D., ABPP, Psychologist ~

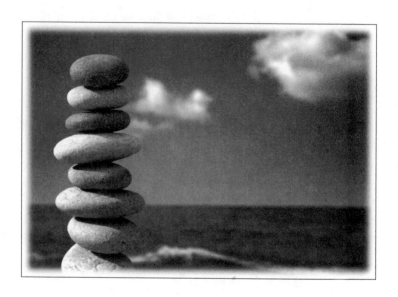

Chapter 1
Stop Being Your Own Worst Enemy

The Multitask Queen at Rest

"**W**hat can I do?" my husband asked as I dropped a torn romaine leaf into the bowl, my fingers shaking as though I'd had too much caffeine. I'd spent the afternoon creating a perfect chicken cacciatore for our dinner guests, who were due to arrive in twenty minutes, and the kitchen was a mess. I paused to rub a knot at the back of my neck that wouldn't budge.

"Here." I passed Gregg a knife and nodded towards the sourdough slices on a cookie sheet. "Butter the bread and sprinkle it with garlic salt." As I rinsed a pan, my eyes slid first to the oven clock and then to the cookie sheet. Gregg was dotting the slices with clumps of butter, tearing the bread in the process.

"Oh for heaven's sake," I said, drying my hands and taking the knife from his hand. "Let me do it." I scooted him out of the way with my hip and deftly spread thin layers of butter to the crusts' edges while reaching for the garlic salt. My temples throbbed and pain held a vice-like grip at the bottom of my skull.

"You're not Mistress of the Universe, you know," Gregg said, leaning against a kitchen counter with his arms crossed.

"Of course I'm not." I winced at the irritation in my voice.

"Then stop acting like it." Gregg took a deep breath. "Look at you. You're stressing and you won't let me help."

I grabbed a napkin to wipe the dampness from my forehead and turned to him. He stepped close and tipped my chin to his face. "Are we having fun yet?" he whispered, making me laugh for the first time that day.

"Are we having fun yet?" We say this to each other when one of us manages to zap the joy from what should be happy events. His reminder showed me how easy it was to fall back to my old ways, those stress-filled days before my meltdown.

While raising three children, I'd crowned myself the Multitask Queen. I was proud of my ability to manage a home, teach full-time, carpool kids to school and activities, cook nightly, help my children with homework, and grade essays until midnight. Sure, I was living a high-stress life, skipping meals and exercise, but I loved the smug feeling of being indispensable. I didn't see that, like Humpty Dumpty, I was primed for a great fall.

I tumbled from that high wall on a Monday afternoon in late spring. In the days before cell phones, my twins, Nick and Kim, were sixth graders and I was an English teacher in another city. I drove in a carpool and wrote the schedule on my calendar faithfully. This particular day had been hectic and I'd skipped lunch, again. At the last bell, I glanced at the calendar and confirmed that my reliable friend, Cathy, had carpool duty. I jammed in a committee meeting and grocery shopping before pulling into the driveway at 4:30. The house was empty. No messages on the phone. No answer at Cathy's house. Where were my children? The other carpool moms didn't answer their phones. How irresponsible of the usually trustworthy Cathy to take the kids somewhere without even a call! At five o'clock my chest hurt and it was getting harder to breathe when Gregg walked through the door.

"Quick," I said. "Get back in the car and drive their school route. Stop by Cathy's to see if anyone's home. I'll wait here in case they show up." I paced the sidewalk, a cold sweat prickling down my back, listening for sirens, willing my children to appear. Magically, two precious figures rounded the corner with backpacks dragging and frowns creasing their faces.

"Where have you been?" I cried, my knees trembling. "I was about to call 911."

"At school," Nick said. "Waiting for you."

"You had carpool today, Mom," Kim said. "We called your classroom and waited forever before the others decided to walk home. Finally we did, too. You're in big trouble with their parents."

I must have written the wrong names in my calendar! Anyone could make this mistake, but I collapsed in a wave of humiliation and guilt, as did the image I'd so carefully fabricated for myself. I stumbled through the rest of the week, unable to make the simplest of decisions. I slept through the weekend, barely able to raise my arms. A doctor confirmed my blood pressure was sky high and I tested positive for anemia. This was my turning point. I had to delegate. My attitude had been that if I didn't do everything myself, it wouldn't be done right. But this left no time to care for myself, or to enjoy the love, happiness and laughter that I was missing.

Now here I was doing it again while preparing for our dinner party, forgetting that our friends only wanted to have a good time with us tonight, not a flawlessly orchestrated dinner. What I had created instead was a perfect recipe for stress.

Our company would arrive in ten minutes and still there was a dirty pot, the table wasn't set, and I wasn't certain if I'd hung a fresh hand towel in the guest bathroom. I looked at Gregg and groaned.

He grinned and said, "If it isn't fun, why do it?"

My eyes surveyed the kitchen. The dinner was ready but the sink was greasy. Gregg picked up a sponge and went to work. "I can handle this."

"I know you can," I said, and my shoulders relaxed a little as I left the room. I thought of that life-altering day long ago and used the memory as a gentle reminder that when I separate myself from tasks and allow others to help, I'm filled with joy instead of stress. In the bathroom I glossed my lips and fluffed my curls. I rubbed a frown line from my brow and studied my face in the mirror. Let go, I admonished the woman in the glass. Accept the way that people do things, and if they're not done your way, so what?

When I walked into the kitchen, the countertops were clean and the dishwasher was loaded. Gregg had lit a candle and the room smelled of fresh pine. I found him leaning against the deck's railing, his back to me, taking in the evening. How grateful I am to have a husband to remind me what is important. When I share chores, I take a major step in eliminating stress. Do I want perfect garlic toast or an evening spent in harmony with my husband and good friends?

I stepped outside and wrapped an arm around Gregg's waist. We watched the setting sun filter through the trees, causing their leaves to sparkle. The tightness in my neck had lessened and my headache was gone. To embrace the moment without a need to control it had set me free.

"I'm having fun now," I said, and meant it.

Gregg squeezed my hand just as the doorbell rang.

~ Sarah Jo Smith ~

It's Not the End of the World

People say I was born standing up and haven't relaxed since. I was a nervous, worried child who often broke out in hives over things other children seemed to take in stride. I was desperately anxious to please people and failure resulted in crushing self-recrimination. When I was five years old and forced to play a difficult piece of music in a piano recital, I was terrified of not playing it well enough. I walked across the stage and became violently ill, putting an end to the recital before I'd played one note. A few years later I was in a school play and the bright footlights blinded me—I walked off the stage and took a nosedive into the audience.

I became so afraid of failing and humiliating myself in front of people that I started avoiding social events. What if I said the wrong thing, spilled something, or made a fool of myself? Something as simple as going to a birthday party would cause me so much stress that I'd hide in my bedroom to keep from going.

Early in my childhood I had decided the universe was an unfriendly place and was out to get me. I exaggerated my problems. I felt overwhelmed and unable to cope. The smallest thing could almost paralyze me.

I avoided people as much as possible because I believed

people were the cause of my stress. Of course, that didn't work. I still had stress in my life but now I was lonely as well.

One day when I was walking to the store, I tripped on the curb and fell onto my knees. An elderly man came to my aid, helped me to my feet and asked if I was hurt.

"No, I think I'm alright. I'm just shaken up and a little embarrassed," I said.

"Well, if you didn't break your knees, then it isn't the end of the world, is it? There's no reason to be embarrassed. We all fall down sometimes. You're okay now," he said, and walked away.

His words rang in my head like a big bell. I'd had a little fall, and yes, I did feel foolish, but I didn't break my knees and it wasn't the end of the world. I realized I didn't have a single problem in my life that would either break my knees or cause the world to come to an end.

Suddenly everything was put into perspective and none of my problems seemed that big anymore. Most of my problems were in the future—very few had to be faced that day or even that week.

I began writing down the things that were troubling me the most: debts, money, family problems, the funny noise under the hood of my car. No matter how big or how small the problem was, I'd write it on a piece of paper and I'd put the piece of paper into a box. On the last day of the month I'd open the box and read the list of my "terrible" problems. I found that almost all of my troubles never happened at all. Or if they had happened, they weren't as bad as I thought they would be or the situation had solved itself without any action from me. The universe didn't need my help. It was a huge relief not to be in charge of the universe anymore. I didn't have to be perfect. It's okay to make mistakes; it's okay to be wrong; it's okay not to have all the answers. It's okay to fail; in fact, it's okay to fail magnificently, gloriously and spectacularly.

Over time, I've put fewer and fewer notes into the box, and some months the box stays empty. It isn't that I don't have problems or that I don't worry or get upset. I still get stressed over things. But I've come to realize that very few things are worth getting upset over, and nothing is ever as bad as I thought it was going to be.

When a new problem comes into my life, I ask myself if it is the end of the world or if it is going to break my knees. If the answer is "no," I write it down and put it in the box.

I'm grateful to that old man; he was only in my life for a minute or two but he changed my life forever. I feel I have cut the stress in my life by eighty percent. I've started going out more, I've made some new friends, and I feel like a new person. I recently played the piano at a party and discovered I'm really bad at it. It's okay—I made everyone laugh and I laughed with them. I'm not afraid of social events or being with people anymore. If I make a mistake or spill something or even fall flat on my face, well, we all fall down sometimes and it's NOT the end of the world!

— April Knight —

Confessions of a Stress Management Consultant

risis is a great teacher. In 1978 my marriage was crumbling, my thirtieth birthday was approaching, and my three-year-old son was begging me to stop smoking. I was desperate, so I booked a massage, unaware that it would crack open a miracle, allowing peace to slide in and change everything.

Back then I didn't know what the word relaxation meant. I was a nurse working in the ICU and I lived on the adrenaline. Death and grief were my constant companions. I drank ten cups of regular coffee a day, exercised little, and consumed lots of sugar and fat. I didn't know what it felt like to be calm, relaxed in my body, connected to my spirit, or have a clear mind that was open, alert, and flexible.

When Mimi, the massage therapist, asked me where I held tension in my body, I didn't know how to answer her. Unless I had a headache or had hurt myself, I never felt my body. Mimi started with soft rhythmic movements of my limbs, and then kneaded my muscles like I kneaded bread dough. Tension evaporated under her touch. I closed my eyes, drifting to a kinder world, one where there were no divorces, where I was cared for, and where the world managed all on its own. Gliding in and out of a reverie, a thought flitted through my consciousness. Was it possible to feel this good and be alive?

After the session I walked across the street and sat in the park. The spring sun was lighting the leaves in the trees. Black squirrels scrambled up and down, occasionally stopping to gaze at me. Tears rolled down my cheeks and I wondered what had happened. I felt whole and connected to everything. In some deep mysterious place within, I made a decision to live a relaxed life. I didn't know what it meant, and I never mentioned my desire to anyone. Looking back, I realize it was the first time I had experienced being present, relaxed, and awake. I wanted more. I saw the possibility of living at one with my body, mind, and spirit, a choice that I had never known before.

A month later I began to study massage with a goal to integrate it into my nursing practice. In the 1970s, therapeutic massage in a clinical setting was unheard of. However, in the middle of the night, when every dose of painkiller had been given and pain still roared, my patients were willing to try anything. I witnessed profound miracles. Soon I added visualization, meditation, and guided imagery to my repertoire, even making audiotapes for patients and families to use on their own.

The more I learned, the more I saw a million ways to actively shift an experience of stress into an opportunity for relaxation. By 1986 I was teaching a range of techniques for pain and stress management in hospitals. By invitation, I spent ten days on a pediatric oncology unit in Paris at the Curie Institute. In 1987 I wrote and self-published the booklet, *Ten Five-Minute Miracles: How to Relax*.

Somewhere along the way, I realized that developing ways to relax had become my spiritual practice. It was also practical. When I slipped on an icy sidewalk and cracked an ankle, I leaned against a building, and using my breath, I put myself into a light meditation. Immediately the pain subsided. Visualizing healing light flowing into my ankle, I did a prayer-mantra, and then walked six blocks to a friend's home. Another time when I came upon a car accident, I was able to quickly teach a breathing technique to the victim, helping to stabilize him until the ambulance came. When I had to have major abdominal surgery, I was equipped mentally, emotionally, physically, and spiritually, and I was discharged four days earlier than expected. When my friend Jenny was dying, I relied on my methods in order to stay present to her pain, her two-year-old's grief, and my own sadness.

A part of me believed that if I practiced long and hard enough, I would have no stress in my life. What I've learned is that I'm a sensitive, vulnerable human being, and that allowing myself to feel and experience all of life opens me even more to stress. I've empowered myself to live fully, not numbing the feelings through old habits such as caffeine, over-eating, smoking, or by focusing on others' drama. I rejoice to bear witness to ups and downs, calm and terror, simple and complex. I love that I can handle big and little stresses, sometimes gracefully and sometimes with anxiety, until I get my bearings. But the awareness to know the difference, and to have that choice, is truly a life-giving miracle.

~ Shirley Dunn Perry ~

Time Out

I had just spent another long, hot, tiring day helping Janet, my best friend, get her house in order. Over the last two weeks, we had cleaned out three rooms, thrown out years of correspondence and files, and organized her medical and financial papers. We'd also boxed half her book collection and bagged three-quarters of her clothes and knickknacks. Since her strength and concentration were waning from the aftermath of radiation treatment for brain cancer, she spent most of her time sitting or lying down while I did the boxing, bagging and carrying stuff downstairs.

By the end of the day, which marked the second full week of the organizing process, I was almost as tired as she was. Her doctor had told her she needed to move out of her two-story house because she wouldn't be able to do the stairs much longer. She had already begun making plans to move in with her ex-husband, who had a main floor bathroom and a living room that would double as her bedroom.

We didn't have much time left. She wanted to get rid of anything she didn't need in case... although we never said the words, there was the underlying fear that once she moved out she might not come back.

I took the last box downstairs and returned to Janet's bedroom. "That's it," I said, rubbing my back, which was protesting all the physical labor. "Everything boxed or bagged is on the front porch waiting for pickup." I gazed around the room. "In the twenty years I've known you, this room has never looked better."

She sighed. "Who knew radiation would turn me into a better housekeeper? Though you're the one doing all the work."

"Hey, that's what a best friend is for." I almost said she could return the favor some day but stopped. Once her cancer had metastasized to her brain, lungs and liver, the chances of her ever being able to do that for me were close to nil. She didn't need me to remind her. I bit my lip to hold the words in and forced a smile. "Just don't tell my mother I did a great job on your house or she'll expect me to do the same on mine."

Knowing my mother, Janet smiled. "You'd better go home or your cats will think you've abandoned them."

"Are you sure you don't want me to stay?" Although I knew her older daughter Denise, who was living with her, would be back soon, I hesitated.

She shook her head and settled herself more comfortably in bed. "Thanks. I mean it. I couldn't have done this without you."

I nodded, still worried about leaving her alone. Then thinking of the forty-five-minute trip home, I let myself out.

A streetcar, a subway, and a bus later, I dragged myself up the stairs and into my house. I dumped my bag in the foyer and crashed on the couch. The last two weeks of helping Janet had used up all my energy. My own house was a mess. Dishes were piled in the sink and on the counters. My living room looked as if a hurricane had torn through it, leaving newspapers, books, papers and files all over the floor, coffee table and chairs. The rest of my house was no better.

I fed the cats. Then, too tired to cook, I ate a cheese and marmalade sandwich, promising myself I would go grocery shopping soon. Promising myself I would start to eat healthy again. Promising myself I would go back on my diet. Promising myself I would... the list went on and on.

As I started to nod off on the couch, I reminded myself I hadn't checked my e-mail since I left for Janet's that morning. I heaved myself off the couch and trudged down the hallway to my office. Closing my eyes to the mess, I turned on the computer.

Damn, there were two e-mails from the moderator of my online writing group. I read the first one and realized I had forgotten to send in the weekly writing exercise for the group. The next e-mail said several of the members had asked what happened to that week's exercise. Joyce, the moderator, was going to wait another hour before sending in an exercise herself. I checked my watch. That was three hours ago.

I zipped off an e-mail. "Joyce, I'm so sorry. I just forgot. I'll do it next week. I promise."

She responded within ten minutes. "Are you sure? I know you're under a lot of stress with Janet being so sick. I can easily get someone else to do it. Maureen and Fiona both volunteered because they know how swamped you are. Or I can do it."

I began typing my response. "No, it's okay. I'll just write it in my calendar." Then I stopped. Sending in the exercise only took a few minutes, but right then I didn't have those few minutes, let alone the energy or mental capacity. Here were three people offering to help and my first response was to refuse, to hold onto yet another commitment. But this time it was a commitment that could easily be done by someone else.

I closed my eyes and took a deep breath.

Erasing what I had typed, I started again. "Joyce, thank you. I know Maureen, Fiona or you will do a wonderful job."

I turned off the computer and returned to the living room. Books and papers were still piled everywhere but I realized that in the grand scheme of things, a neat living room, kitchen or office weren't even on the same list as helping a friend. The mess would still be there tomorrow and the day after and the day after that. I would get to it when I could.

Right now, however, I needed a time out from responsibilities and expectations, mostly my own. I dug into a pile of books, found one that looked like a fun read, and settled in for a relaxing evening.

— Harriet Cooper —

Stop Being Your Own Worst Enemy

Introduction

Have you ever wondered why you feel so discombobulated when you try to do too many things at once? It's because you overload your neuro-circuitry and everything in your brain goes awry. A bottleneck occurs in your frontal cortex, the part of the brain responsible for focus, attention and working memory among other things, so information no longer squeezes through to other parts of the brain. An increase of neural firing is desperately needed, but instead, activity fizzles. Worse, your brain tries to divide and conquer. Activity that normally runs through both halves of the brain at once — presumably to strengthen the connection between thought and task — splits instead, with one half veering to the left hemisphere, the other traveling right. Instead of doubling, brain activity cuts in half. Instead of accomplishing everything, you often wind up accomplishing nothing. I think any of the multitasking mavens who shared their stories in this chapter would agree.

Modern Overload

Multitasking, the art and skill of doing more than one thing at a time, is something we all love to do. Ok, maybe some of us don't love it, but we think it's a requirement given the demands of today's world. At work you can't just focus on writing a report. You've also got to keep checking your e-mail and pick up the phone every time it rings, which is often. Then, e-mail follows you home, stealing chunks of focus away from cooking dinner, reviewing homework and chatting with your spouse. Text messages and two or three different phones also compete for your attention. In case you're not on overload yet, TV, iPad, Facebook, Twitter, YouTube and a mind-boggling array of other social media sources add to the multimedia din. But, as the Multitasking Queen story illustrates, the idea of multitasking predates the era of electronic and digital overload.

Thanks to the proliferation of technology and gadgets, we've begun to multitask at insane levels. Observational studies have found that the average computer user at work switches between windows or checks e-mail an average of 37 times an hour. More than 90 percent of workers say they make or take work-related communications outside of the office, including during vacations, according to a recent Lexmark International study. Nearly 75 percent say they stay "switched on" during weekends with 20 percent admitting they interrupt social engagements for work reasons.

We all assume we can handle this amount of multitasking and in fact, many of us think we're pretty good at it. Actually we're pretty bad at it. One study by researchers at the University of California at Irvine monitored interruptions among office workers and found they take an average of twenty-five minutes to recover from disruptions such as phone calls or answering e-mail before returning to their original task. The heaviest-hitting multitaskers have the most trouble focusing and shutting out irrelevant information so they can even bring one task to successful completion.

This Is Your Brain on Multitasking

Scientists estimate that each time you switch from one task to another you more than double the time it takes to complete either task. As a result, performance quality takes a nosedive. You weaken the memory of what you were doing, which leads to shallow learning. Even after you cease multitasking, splintered thinking and lack of focus can persist.

At its worst, multitasking can have dangerous consequences: We all know by now that drivers who text or talk on a cell phone show the same level of impairment as drivers who are legally drunk. At its best, constant task switching and attentional flip flopping cut into work and family time and stifle creativity. Would Sir Isaac Newton have dreamed up his breakthrough ideas on gravity if he'd been yakking on a cell phone while also texting and surfing the Net rather than sitting in quiet contemplation under an apple tree?

And multitasking really does ratchet up stress levels. The brain responds to task-and-information overload by pumping out adrenaline and other stress hormones that contribute to the feelings of agitation and edginess. Long-term exposure to these hormones can lead to classic stress symptoms like headaches, stomach aches and sleep disturbances. One report by the Institute of the Future in California found that 71 percent of white-collar workers feel stressed about the amount of information they must process and act on while doing business; 60 percent feel overwhelmed. The more overworked an employee, the more likely he is to make mistakes, feel angry with his employers and resent his colleagues. Those with higher stress levels also report more symptoms of clinical depression and poorer health.

Stop the Madness

There is evidence that multitasking is a hard habit to break because it mimics some aspects of addiction. Some people need their fix of constant data flow and task jumping so much they become dependent upon it. As a result they develop shorter attention spans and lose their ability to complete activities that require deep concentration. Their desks become littered with half completed projects, they have difficulty thinking clearly and they feel like they're drowning in a pool of unfinished business. There's even a term for this narcotic-like effect: pseudo-attention deficit disorder.

But extreme multitasking doesn't have to be a way of life. If your goal is to reduce stress and increase productivity, it pays to adopt a philosophy of single-tasking. Single-tasking — now there's a word for the information age! — means slowing down, doing less, and turning off the information spigot, at least sometimes. As you sit here reading — and perhaps also responding to texts and instant messages that pop up on your computer screen—you may think this is easier said than done. I can tell you it's harder for some people to do than others.

A good first step is to make a list of everything you need to get done. In a way this is what April Knight did by slipping notes into a box each month. Go through the list to evaluate whether every item truly needs to be there and toss out anything that isn't important, can be delegated or doesn't truly require your immediate involvement. Once you've got your final list, put the mundane, rote tasks aside for the moment and prioritize the bigger items from most to least important using a 1-10 or A-Z designation.

Now structure your day so that you spend the first 15-30 minutes banging out the mindless need-to-dos like responding to e-mails and signing off on forms. After that, focus on the highest priority task for an uninterrupted, designated block of time that lasts at least 30 minutes or a predetermined amount of time to sufficiently address it. Allot as much time as you need for each task, and only that task, until it's completed or you've reached a predetermined target goal for progress. It helps to underestimate what you think you'll be able to accomplish so you don't get discouraged or feel like you're falling behind.

Multitasking junkies may experience actual withdrawal symptoms when they try going cold turkey to slow themselves down. You're apt to find a gradual approach more palatable. For instance, see how you feel when you shut off your cell phone in 30-minute increments and check your e-mail only once per hour rather than every time an e-mail pops up. Once you can tolerate that level of disconnect, consider extending your technology blackouts for longer intervals.

If your desk is a mess, clean it up; a less cluttered desk equals a less cluttered mind. You'll waste less time if everything is kept in a designated place. Keep your door closed if you have one, or ask your co-workers to check in only at appointed times unless there's an emergency.

At home, set limits on how often you check up on work. You might, for example, delegate the first hour you come home and the last hour before bedtime as technology-free time to help you relax and savor the separation of work and family. I strongly believe family meals should be sacred, with no texting, answering phones or watching TV allowed. Leave your cell phone at home for short trips to the market or dry cleaners to help you get more comfortable with the idea of being unplugged. Or like Newton, find an apple tree to sit under and just think. Who knows what bright ideas might pop into your brain when you give it a break from multitasking madness?

The Power of No

People with 15-20 major items on their daily to-do list either haven't sorted their priorities carefully or they're seriously over-committed. I think over commitment is partly caused by a propensity for multitasking; it too is epidemic and causes needless stress. When I have a patient who is drowning in obligations and responsibilities we explore how he or she got there.

Over-obligators generally fall into one of two categories:

They're either compulsive people pleasers who fear disappointing or angering other people, or they're poor time managers who have a warped sense of what it takes to get stuff done.

People pleasers need to dial down the guilt. They must get comfortable with the word "no" and learn to reframe their criteria for saying "yes." Before agreeing to take on a responsibility, do a cost-benefit analysis to decide whether or not it's worth your time. I don't mean you should only be saying yes to things that make you money, but when you sign on for something you prefer not to do, you are in actuality saying no to your own priorities.

Time mismanagers need to get real and do an honest assessment of what they can reasonably take on. Not every offer that comes your way is a good use of your time or feeds your priorities. And since we are speaking of priorities as they relate to both people pleasers and time mismanagers, do you know what yours are? Have some clear ideas of what you value most. Whether that's family time, career, charity work, exercise, learning—or yes, even money—keep in mind what's most important to you every time you respond to a request. This will help you dispassionately decide what deserves your attention.

I do realize that saying no takes some practice and may not be easy for you, especially if you're used to saying yes reflexively. So I've got some tips for you.

Keep track of how many times each week you now say yes and you wish you hadn't. Surprised at how often that is? I had one client who had serious political aspirations but always complained about not having enough time to pull her campaign together. She was a people pleaser and an incurable yes woman. Her unwanted yes count was astonishing; it wasn't difficult to determine what sucked away her potential planning time.

Saying no is a skill you need to practice. The more you do it the easier it gets. No need to be defensive, ungracious or apologetic when turning down a request: a polite but firm "thanks, but no thanks" usually does the trick. You don't owe anyone an explanation for your decision, but if it helps, come up with a well-crafted stock reply you can pull out whenever necessary. You might beg off for genuine health reasons, family commitments, or work obligations. I sometimes use humor to lessen the blow.

If someone is insistent and won't take no for an answer, tell them you'll think about it; you can always write them a polite and final note saying no at a later date. Stepping out of a pressure-filled situation gives you some time to think and reaffirm your priorities. Plus it's less stressful to turn someone down when you're not face-to-face.

If you'd really like to help out but it's too much of a commitment at the moment, you can offer up something less. You might say, "I can't do this right now, but I can donate such and such…" This allows you to be involved without full engagement. Honestly, most opportunities that come your way are interesting on some level.

The biggest surprise for yes people is that the world doesn't come to an end when you say no. You won't become a pariah or the object of derision because you graciously declined an invitation to become involved. There may be some lingering guilt at first but I promise you this rarely lasts long. There are only so many hours in a day. Doing more of what you want to do and doing less in general will make you a happier person in the long run.

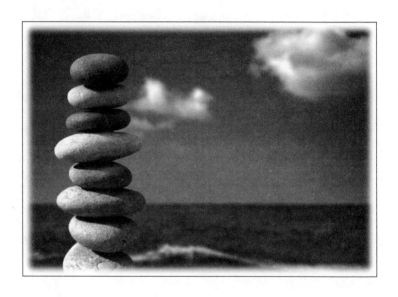

Chapter 2
Triumph Over Tragedy

Love and Music

I stood on the front porch of the old Varner-Hogg Plantation house in West Columbia, Texas, gazing into the eyes of my soon-to-be husband Anthony. As the minister asked me to promise "for better or worse," thunder rumbled loudly from the overcast sky. Was it a warning or a promise?

I'd already been through "the worse." Surely nothing but "the better" was in our future. In the past sixteen months I had gone through a divorce, lost my job, moved, and watched helplessly as my mother rapidly succumbed to breast cancer that had spread too far before it was discovered.

I'd spent as much time as I could with her, and after her struggle was over, with my dad as he tried to adjust to life without his beautiful wife. He had decided to sell their home and live life on the road in a travel trailer, traversing the country to spend time with relatives. He had been in West Columbia for a week or so before the wedding, getting to know my new husband and doing dad stuff like fixing things around the house, making sure the car was in top shape, etc. A few days after the wedding he would head to my brother's house for a while, then off on his cross-country trek.

Anthony and I spent our wedding night in nearby Galveston, and came home the next afternoon.

Monday morning I was back at work when Dad called me.

"I'm so cold," he said. "I have the heater all the way up and I can't get warm."

It was in the seventies outside.

I left work and finally convinced him to let me take him to the emergency room. Anthony had arrived to wait with me by the time the doctor came out with the diagnosis. Dad had a huge tumor in his colon. The tumor had sapped his blood supply, which made him anemic and accounted for the inability to get warm. He needed surgery right away.

They removed the tumor, and told us that after a period of recovery he was going to have to go through chemo.

Okay, our married life was not starting out on the "better" side, but I was so glad I had Anthony to love and lean on as we nursed Dad through this.

Dad was in his first month of chemotherapy when I scheduled a visit to my ob-gyn. I'd had a mammogram just a few months after mom died—my first one. It showed no abnormalities. But lately I had noticed that my left nipple was beginning to sink in, and I'd heard that was not a good sign.

The doctor sent me right away to the hospital for a mammogram and a sonogram.

One of the hardest things I've ever had to do was stand in the hospital parking lot that afternoon and call my husband of five months to tell him I had been diagnosed with breast cancer and needed a mastectomy.

So here we were, Dad going through his chemotherapy and me recovering from surgery and then beginning chemotherapy, too. We called it our father-daughter bonding experience.

Anthony was working, taking care of two chemo patients and my kids, too. He never once complained, but no matter how hard he tried to hide it I knew he would break down now and then.

The stress of trying to handle what Dad was going through and what I was going through was bad enough, but to see what it was doing to my husband sometimes drove me over the edge. I knew he loved me, but even love wouldn't have been enough for most men. He deserved so much more.

It was the radiation nurse who gave me a solution, not for changing things, but for dealing with it all.

"Spend time every day in music therapy," she said. "It doesn't have to be relaxation music. Just go in a quiet place, all alone, and listen to anything you want."

I almost always had music or something going on around me, so I didn't see how that was going to be helpful, but one afternoon when I didn't know how I was going to keep going I went in the bedroom, crawled under the covers, put on my earphones and turned on the CD player.

I played Billy Joel and Paul Simon over and over, until I eventually felt strong enough to get up and face life again with a smile. The small changes my daily music time made in my attitude had a ripple effect on my husband, and I could sense the tension lessening for him, too.

Since that time, when the kids, or grandkids, or things at work, or even the recurrence of the cancer some ten years later, have tried to knock me down, I know that a little time alone with music will help refresh me. I can always tell if it's been too long since I've spent time alone in a cocoon of my favorite tunes.

There have been plenty of times in the twenty years since our wedding day when it seems as though the "for worse" side of our vows has more than overshadowed the "for better" side, but each time we've come through it even stronger.

A whole lot of love, and a little music, is all it takes.

~ Teena Maenza ~

A Natural
Approach
to Stress

As my husband and I walked around the lake, our pace was significantly slower than many of the joggers and cyclists who sailed past us. We made our way to a bench nestled in the shade of a giant cottonwood tree. Sitting there, we paused to take a breath and allow ourselves to slow down and enjoy the beauty around us.

We laughed at the antics of an indignant squirrel as he made it clear that he did not want us anywhere nearby. He chirped and fussed, racing up and down the tree, seemingly annoyed at our venture into his domain.

Across the lake a small island held a stand of trees with numerous nests of egrets and cormorants. As the beautiful birds swooped in and landed on the branches, I found myself caught up in the peace of our surroundings, and it was a welcome peace.

Only a few months before, my husband had been diagnosed with acute myeloid leukemia. Our lives had changed in an instant. As one might imagine, the stress during that time was tremendous.

My husband was rushed into induction chemotherapy,

which placed him in remission. Another round of chemotherapy followed, with the hope of keeping him in remission until doctors could find a match among his brothers and sisters for a stem cell transplant. When his sister was determined to be an excellent match, we prepared ourselves for the move to a hospital in a neighboring city for the transplant.

I would travel back and forth to be with my husband, sometimes staying the night, sometimes heading home for the evening to be with my adult children. But then, the week before he was to enter the hospital, we received news that made me feel as if the floor below me was falling away. In addition to his time in the hospital, my husband would need to stay nearby in a hotel for two to two-and-a-half months following his release. There were good reasons. If an infection or other problem developed, he would need to be able to get to the hospital in thirty minutes or less.

Our home was an hour's drive away on good days. During heavy traffic times it could be much more. How could we possibly make this work? My stress level started to rise.

Now don't misunderstand me. Stress was nothing new to us. As the parents of three adult children with special needs, we knew the effects of stress all too well. Yet through our experiences, we had forged a good and happy life. Our adult children lived with us in our home. They were quite independent, but I worried about how our new challenges would put that independence to the test, as I moved away to become my husband's full-time caregiver.

Dear friends and family came forward to help, some

spending periods of time with the kids in our absence, others driving one son back and forth to work. We developed a plan to move through this challenge. Yet in spite of all the plans, I still found myself feeling stressed and anxious, not only about my husband, but about my family at home.

Many helpful suggestions were offered by caring people. "Make sure you find some time for yourself," counseled one friend. "Take lots of walks and read lots of books," recommended another.

After my husband's transplant, I was invited to participate in a research study exploring stress among caregivers. As part of the study I used a machine that monitored my respiration. I would strap the cloth band around my diaphragm and follow the prompts playing through the headphones. "Breathe in, breathe out," the gentle, recorded voice told me. "Try to structure your breathing. Relax."

The daily breathing exercises did help me to relax. The walks and times spent within the pages of well-loved books also helped, but as the days went by I recognized that the greatest stress reliever for me was found in nature.

Whether it was pausing to watch a beautiful sunset, seeing bunnies playing on the grass below our hotel window, or just feeling the evening breeze on my face, there were things all around me that replenished my soul and eased my stress. Those things helped me see God's hand not only in my own life but in everything.

As my husband and I sat on the park bench and watched that silly squirrel, I breathed deeply and smiled. I was grateful for a moment's peace and for a greater appreciation of the natural stress relievers that were everywhere.

～ Jeannie Lancaster ～

In Cuffs

I pulled into the local grocery store parking lot. Did I want to go in? No! It had only been three and a half weeks since my sister had died unexpectedly. On the morning of her sixty-third birthday she was literally dancing with delight over her flowers, cards and balloons. That evening she had dinner with friends. Then about 10 p.m., as she slept, her heart simply stopped. And my sister, nine years my senior, was gone.

I was stunned. Grief and sadness filled me. I couldn't sleep. During the day I began to feel pressure in my chest and experience shortness of breath. On top of those physical alarms I wasn't sure from one moment to the next if I would be buoyed up with some lovely memory of my sister, or capsized into an ocean of tears. Through it all, my chest felt tight and my heart pounded. I needed help. I called the nurse practitioner.

At the nurse practitioner's I explained the situation between bouts of tears. I asked her to take my blood pressure. I said, "I know it's high." I had never had high blood pressure before, but I was correct. She kindly assured me it was understandable with all of the stress in my life. She said I needed to have three consecutive blood pressure readings, however, to make a correct diagnosis. I was given a sleep aid, anti-anxiety medication, and instructions to go to the closest Schnucks, a grocery store chain, to use their free blood pressure machine to chart the next two readings.

The day after, I went to Schnucks. As I walked in, I surveyed the store to see if there was anyone I knew. I did not want to break down in the store. I made my way to the back as inconspicuously as possible to where the blood pressure machine sat in wait. As I approached, my heart beat faster. My reading was going to be high. I cuffed myself and hit the button. I took deep breaths and silently told the machine I was okay. But the machine said it was high. So I decided a nice little stroll through the store would be good; perhaps a little shopping would keep my mind off things. I looked at greeting cards, movies; I went by the bakery and the summer clearance aisle. But pressure reading number two remained steady.

This pattern was repeated the next day. This time I knew the first reading would be the worst. Mindful of cameras above watching my every move, I went back and forth from the blood pressure machine to wheeling the cart around the store so I wouldn't look like an idiot fascinated with the piece of machinery over by the pharmacy. But reading number three from the evil cuff said I was still high, so I put the call in to the nurse.

After three days on the blood pressure medicine I felt tightness in my chest once again. That's when I found myself in the Schnucks parking lot one more time. I did deep breathing. I got out of the car and walked through the automatic doors and back to my nemesis. By the time I got to the blood pressure machine I was so worked up that when I saw my numbers (Stage 1 hypertension), I decided to ask the pharmacist if I was going to have a heart attack on the spot. If so, this was okay. Next to a doctor's office or firehouse, a pharmacy was probably the best place to be. It would be even better if I announced it ahead of time. I approached the pharmacist and explained my situation. She must have seen my panic. She assured me that I was fine, and said "Call your doctor if you have questions." As I turned away, a young woman who had been a captive audience to my drama smiled at me and said, "You're not going to die." With that I slunk away, embarrassed and mad at myself for getting so worked up.

So once again I shopped. I looked at more greeting cards and put six of them in my cart. I walked down the summer clearance aisle, which I now had memorized. I grabbed some milk and some rather large bags of Cracker Jacks. And as covertly as possible I crept back to the machine to read my fate. The cuff gave me the news: the numbers had dropped but not enough.

The nurse practitioner got me in the next day. Again I cried. I told her how the blood pressure machine had pulled at me, like a moth to the flame. I had become obsessed. I thought I would pass out or die right there at Schnucks. I understood it was feeding on itself, the blood pressure devil back by the pharmacy, and my sense of panic. But I simply could not help myself.

Then came the time for a reading, and she wrapped the loathed cuff around my arm. I took a deep breath. I heard the push-push sound as yet another evil cuff inflated and the whoosh-whoosh as it deflated. Then the Velcro ripped apart and she announced with a smile, "Your blood pressure is good!"

I laughed with relief.

She said, "You know, there is a lady who has high blood pressure who comes to this office. For ten years she's carried a cuff in her purse and she has one at home.... I think she has at least three. Once she was in a restaurant, started feeling bad and took her pressure right there. It's taken us all this time, but I think we've finally weaned her off the cuff. My advice to you, Mary, is to stay away from the blood pressure machine. Don't go. You're fine. You just have some stressful issues going on, and you have medications to help you through temporarily. What you're going through is difficult and life-changing. But you're going to be okay."

I felt the tension leave my body. The pressure left my chest. I said, "Jeanne, thank you! I already feel so much better just having talked to you. I won't go back to that blood pressure machine. I promise. But Jeanne... they're sure gonna miss me at Schnucks."

— Mary Hughes —

Triumph Over Tragedy

Introduction

You may associate "loss" with the death of someone close to you but there are many other types of loss too, like the breakup of a marriage, being laid off from a job or surviving some catastrophic event. Loss is an evitable part of life. Everyone experiences it at some point.

With loss comes grief. It's often said there are five stages of grief but from my experience, a lot of people grieve in waves. (For the record, the commonly cited stages of grief originally theorized by Elisabeth Kübler-Ross are: denial, anger, bargaining, depression, and acceptance.) Some people feel emotions immediately, especially within the first few hours after a tragedy. For others, the surge of emotions hits them at a funeral, a memorial service or even when a special song comes on the radio months later.

What emotions are appropriate to grief? Sadness, anger, relief, guilt, despair—or nothing at all. Emotions can run deeper than you ever imagined or stir together in ways you find confusing and distressing. You may have trouble focusing and feel no interest in things you normally enjoy.

All of these are expected emotional reactions to loss. And, although expressions of sorrow vary from person to person and culture to culture, everyone—whether they are a tribesman from Papua New Guinea or a saleswoman from San Francisco, California—experiences the heartache of bereavement in some fashion. It's part of the human experience, and a stressful one at that. In fact, the first six events on the Holmes and Rahe stress scale are related to loss, with the death of a loved one topping the list.

Because mind and body are linked, grief can take a physical toll. Mary Hughes learned this when her blood pressure shot up after her beloved sister passed away. Studies on the effects of stress show how it can trigger a flood of brain chemicals into your nervous system, causing a flight or fight response that makes your heart race and your blood pressure rise. One study recently commissioned by the American Heart Association tracked the heart rates of bereaved patients and found that they experienced twice the number of rapid heartbeat episodes as usual in the weeks immediately following their loss. Their average resting heart rates were also significantly higher than normal for at least six months following the death of a loved one.

It's also well established that the stress of grief compromises the immune system. Additionally, those experiencing grief can suffer a variety of symptoms such as exhaustion, sleep disruptions, heart palpitations, shortness of breath, headaches, recurrent infections, high blood pressure, loss of appetite, overeating, digestive upsets, hair loss, and disordered menstrual cycles. Pre-existing chronic conditions like arthritis, eczema and asthma can get worse or flare up for the first time. Someone in a state of grief may be less apt to care for himself so there's a greater chance for health vulnerabilities.

Holmes and Rahe Stress Inventory

Instructions: The following scale was developed by Holmes and Rahe to investigate the relationship between events which can happen to us, stress and susceptibility to illness. Look over the events listed below. Mark the item if it has happened to you within the last twelve months. (You can multiply it by the number of times if you want to really check!)

Event	Points	Yes/No	Score
1. Death of a spouse	100		
2. Divorce	72		
3. Marital separation	65		
4. Death of a close family member	63		
5. Personal injury or illness	53		
6. Marriage	50		
7. Marital reconciliation	45		
8. Change in health of family member	44		
9. Pregnancy	40		
10. Gain of new family member	39		
11. Job Change	38		
12. Change in financial status	37		
13. Death of a close friend	36		
14. Increase in arguments with significant other	35		
15. Mortgage or loan of major purchase (home, etc.)	31		
16. Foreclosure of mortgage or loan	30		

Continued on next page

17. Change in responsibilities of your job	29	____	____
18. Son or daughter leaving home	29	____	____
19. Trouble with in-laws	29	____	____
20. Outstanding personal achievement	28	____	____
21. Spouse begins or stops work outside the home	26	____	____
22. Revision of personal habits	24	____	____
23. Trouble with boss	23	____	____
24. Change in work hours or conditions	20	____	____
25. Change in residence	20	____	____
26. Change in sleeping habits	16	____	____
27. Change in eating habits	15	____	____
28. Vacation	13	____	____
29. Christmas	12	____	____
30. Minor violations of the law	11	____	____
Total			____

0-149 no significant problem
150-199 mild stress 35% chance of illness or health change
200-299 moderate stress 50% chance of illness or health change
300+ major stress 80% chance of illness or health change.

Reprinted from Journal of Psychosomatic Research, Volume 11, Thomas H. Holmes & Richard H. Rahe, The social readjustment rating scale, Pages 213-218, Copyright 1967, with permission from Elsevier.

Even the risk of your own death is greater after you experience a loss. This fact was established as far back as 1969 when a large study of widowers famously reported a bereaved spouse's chance of dying in the first six months after losing a partner was 40% higher than average. Numerous other investigations into "death by broken heart" have yielded similar findings.

Different Forms of Grief

Feelings of loss can be experienced before the actual loss has occurred. Anticipatory grief can be felt just as deeply as grief after a loss. Frequently people use this time to tie up loose ends, seek forgiveness and say, "I love you." It's an experience that can be painful for sure, yet also cathartic and a significant step in the grief process.

Sudden loss can bring on unique emotional experiences, too. You're given no time to prepare when tragedy strikes so, even if you intellectually comprehend what has happened, it can take a while for emotions to catch up. In my experience, I've seen that this surreal feeling can last a lot longer than you might imagine. For example, it's not uncommon for someone who has been laid off unexpectedly to feel fine at first, only to have despair set in several weeks later.

Unresolved grief transpires when a loss goes unexplained, there are confusing issues surrounding the loss or your grief is not generally accepted as legitimate. Losing a pet is a perfect example of this. You may be closer to your dog, cat or ferret than anyone else in the world, but if she passes away you're expected to go to work the next day as if nothing has happened. Others may be clueless about how deep the bonds between pet and owner run, and as a result they may not rally around you or relate to how badly you hurt on the inside.

When depression and other symptoms last longer than a year, some mental health professionals refer to it as complicated grief. Emotions that don't lessen over time or still feel as fresh as if the loss just happened may be pegged as a chronic condition. Certainly the intensity of grief can vary according to the type of loss. As a professional I become concerned when grief never occurs or if it occurs for a protracted period of time. I also monitor to see if grief interferes with life in a debilitating way. In these instances, it's possible that something besides grief may be going on and it should be investigated professionally. That said, I believe it's artificial to impose a deadline on feelings. I take into consideration how well a person is able to function in his daily life before labeling his grief with a diagnosis. However, it's true that healthy people usually do feel their grief gradually subside over time—or at least learn to manage it in a healthy way.

I took the time to define some types of grief because I want you to understand how feelings of loss can take on many forms and still be considered normal. It's not uncommon to cycle through several types of grief and multiple mourning periods. (However, some grief responses are cause for worry and for a mourning period that lasts too long or too intensely, I strongly suggest seeking professional help.) No matter what, the important thing is to have solid coping mechanisms at your disposal to get you through the tough times.

Getting Past and Moving On

All cultures have rituals related to loss, especially the death of a loved one. Such rituals can be religious, cultural, community based or family oriented. They're designed to honor the life of a person or event but they're also meant to help those grieving the loss move towards closure and healing. This is why most cultures hold some type of funeral ceremony shortly after a death.

Rituals related to loss can be especially comforting in the first few days after a tragedy because it gives people who were touched by it a structured way to spend time together, share memories and support one another. Some cultures have designated mourning periods that go beyond the funeral event. In Judaism the practice of "sitting Shiva" involves visitation to the family of the deceased for seven days after the burial. Catholics have a wake where everyone brings food, swaps stories and sometimes even tells jokes about the departed. Some religions hold a service on the one-year anniversary of a death.

One typical response during these events is to cry. For some, it's just too soon or too hard to put their sadness on display. Men in particular have been "trained" not to let emotions leak out in public so they put up a stoic front even when they feel crushed on the inside. It's also not unusual to see people smiling and laughing at a service. When it comes to discussions about death, I've heard people make jokes about "buying the farm," "kicking the bucket" and "biting the dust." Often these remarks aren't meant to be disrespectful but are rather an attempt to humorously diffuse the stress of intense emotions—though I must say they're not always successful. The main point is that being around other mourners can be a comfort and a reminder that some factors in life will stay the same.

If it helps you feel better, create your own ritual to mark a loss. I have one patient who lost a dearly loved aunt but was unable to get to her funeral because of distance and expense. He wanted to do something to mark her passing—so he took his family to an amusement park. This may seem insensitive, but riding the rides at the local theme park were his favorite memories of his adventurous aunt. It was a fitting tribute he says she would have loved. What better way to honor her memory?

After the designated mourning period, you may still feel a strong urge to reach out for support. You may find it comforting to share stories about what is now missing from your life. If you feel the need to communicate your feelings, I urge you to find a way to do it. You can talk to friends and family, join a support group, or see a therapist or grief counselor. Pour your heart out into a journal, a poem, artwork, or a song if that's easier than sharing deep personal emotions with others. You can listen to music too; Teena Maenza did that and as her story reveals, this has helped her through some tough times. It doesn't really matter so long as your need to share is being met.

On the other hand you may be someone who prefers to stay busy to keep your mind off things. That's fine too if that's what you need to do, though I find at some point emotions need to be expressed and released. If you hold them in for too long, they tend to leak out at surprising times and in surprising ways. You might consider channeling your stress and grief into something positive like planting a tree, creating a foundation or raising money for a cause related to your loss. One of the best ways to manage bad feelings is by doing something good.

However you grieve, remember those left behind. That includes you. Take care of yourself in small but strategic ways. Take a walk, sit on a bench, watch a silly squirrel. Because grief can be so physically taxing, make it a point to eat right, sleep well and get some exercise. Besides helping you stave off sickness, all of these things help boost mood too.

I know sometimes it can be hard to get motivated enough to care. Grief can leave you lethargic and disinterested in life. That's why I emphasize covering the basics of good health rather than committing to a complete lifestyle overhaul. Just as it makes sense to avoid making major decisions right after you've suffered a loss, it's probably not the time to start training for a marathon or to follow a radical diet.

What Not to Do

When you're paralyzed by the depression and stress of a loss, it can seem easier to withdraw from the world. Dropping out of life won't help you heal. Spend some time alone if you must—wanting private time to grieve is understandable—but don't lose touch with the social and spiritual connections that can be so pivotal to recovery. Though it may feel like going through the motions when you stick to your routine, do it anyway. Go to work, attend classes and have dinner with friends; these are the things that will help you find your groove again.

If you've been down in the dumps for months on end and

still can't seem to get back on track, consider seeing a professional mental health expert. Feeling sad is okay so long as your emotions don't overwhelm you for long periods of time. Counseling with a professional therapist can help because it allows you to talk about your loss and express those deep feelings, especially if you feel hopeless or feel like ending your own life. If you'd like to talk to a therapist and you're not sure where to begin, ask your doctor, clergy, trusted friend, or a human resources representative at work. They're usually a good source for therapy referrals.

Well-meaning friends and family may tell you that you need to "move on" after a loss. Unfortunately, this sort of advice can backfire, leading you to believe your grief is somehow inappropriate. We all grieve differently—on our own schedules—and no matter what anyone else thinks, there is no right or wrong way to grieve as long as how you grieve is safe. If you don't like the idea of moving on, then maybe the idea of "keeping on" is easier to accept.

Prolonged and inappropriate grief can lead you to try harmful behaviors in order to ease your pain. Engaging in self-destructive activities will only make you feel worse. Drinking, drugs or hurting your body in other ways to escape the pain of a loss are delay tactics for dealing with sorrow. They temporarily mask your pain but make it harder to heal in the long run because they prolong grief. These are instances when you should be consulting a therapist.

Going forward and healing from grief doesn't mean forgetting about what you lost. It's not a sin to enjoy life again. And how long it takes until you start to feel better isn't a measure of how much you loved what you now grieve. With time, the loving support of family and friends, and your own positive actions, you may find ways to cope with even the deepest loss and come out of it stronger than ever.

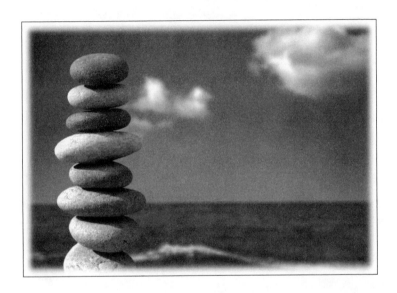

Chapter 3
Killer Jobs—
Stress and the
Workplace

Stress Points

"Doctor, Doctor, come quickly—a confused patient has just driven away in our ambulance!" I rushed out to see the ambulance disappearing south on the road towards the dangerous pass. Quickly we dispatched a second vehicle, with two regular hospital drivers in it, to chase after the precious ambulance. "That's worth five stars," I ticked off in my mind. I had already collected three stars that day from arguments between key members of my hospital staff. It was going to be a top day for a crisis score.

There seem to be an inexhaustible supply and an infinite variety of crises that reach the superintendent's desk in an African mission hospital. As that superintendent, I quickly found that I had to devise a way to withdraw a little from these frequent problems, or the stress could cause burnout. I could not afford to get emotionally involved whenever the smooth running of the hospital was threatened. For this reason I developed a scoring system by which each new problem could be graded from one (mild) to five (catastrophic), taking into account the nature and implications of each occurrence. I could then keep a running tally and see whether the day would break any record as the score rose. While this didn't make me relish new challenges, at least it provided a harmless game that kept my feet firmly on the ground.

By analyzing problems in this way I could keep cool when threats appeared and view the issues from outside my own emotions. This helped me to plan solutions dispassionately.

Unfortunately staff shortages are the norm in mission hospitals. This meant that I had to take my full share of clinical duties as well as administrative tasks. Rounds in the children's ward were an emotionally draining experience. Malnutrition leaves the kids vulnerable to every infection and their resistance is poor, meaning the mortality rate is high.

Every few nights there would be call duties, which meant a full round of the hospital to check on critical patients, and then often being called to new patients in casualty or a patient who had deteriorated suddenly.

I found that the only way I could control the stress generated by the workload and the constant calls to help desperately ill patients was to free my mind completely of all the current problems when I returned home to my wife and family. I would turn to other interests the moment I got back and forget the problem patients whom I had been assessing. I found that I was able to do this so well that when a nurse called to say something like: "Doctor, that ill patient in the female ward has got worse," I would not know it was the seriously ill typhoid case until the nurse reminded me of the details. Then it would be clear and I could rush to the ward and prescribe the necessary treatment. My home thus became a fortress against the daily stress.

And the missing ambulance? An hour after the vehicles had roared out of the hospital, they both returned safely with the hospital drivers in control and the confused patient seated quietly in a passenger seat. The report I received was that the patient had stopped the ambulance neatly at a viewpoint in the pass, and was found standing and admiring the fine view. He quietly returned to join the driver for his return trip to the hospital. I firmly believe it was worth the five stars I gave it!

~ John McCutcheon ~

And a Little Child Shall Lead Them

The Borders bookstore where I've worked the past four years will be closing soon, and it has been a very difficult first week of liquidation sales. Our store has wonderful employees who are close like family, and we feel as if we are in mourning. But there's no time to grieve because customers have descended upon us like locusts, tearing our store apart in search of bargains. We are working as many hours as allowed by the liquidators, yet can't keep up with the mess. What's most painful is that the days we all loved are over. No more taking the time to help someone find a book, offering a suggestion or, what I loved most, my weekly children's story time.

I had a big crowd at story time last week. After I announced it was the last one, the parents thanked me, then stood and applauded. The tears I'd been shedding quietly and alone at home during my sleepless nights finally came to the store. We were all sad, and no one wanted to leave.

Yesterday I discovered a young girl in the children's area—my beloved area of the store—carefully going through the children's chapter books and sorting them, alphabetizing them, trying to put them back in order. I watched her for a few minutes, not sure what she was doing at first. But when it was clear, I was truly touched. I had given up on that area and had, myself, put the books in any order, just to have them off the floor. I went to get some leftover giveaway books and a store employee lanyard for her. When I returned, the young girl's mother was sitting on the floor waiting patiently as her daughter continued to work. I told her what a wonderful daughter she's raising and how deeply moved I was by her efforts, and presented her with my small tokens. The girl put on the lanyard and continued working, eventually finishing that area and moving onto another.

I felt like I had witnessed a small miracle. I am not a religious person, but I thought of the phrase "and a little child shall lead them." That little girl inspired me to take more care with the books I needed to shelve. That small bit of normalcy helped me feel much less stressed. Now every time I'm in the children's area, I remember her and smile.

I realized how important it is to remember what I will miss from my work, so I started a list. I thought about why each employee was special to me and wrote it down, like James's inspirational leadership, Sandy's effervescence, how David makes the animal puppets talk, and even the way Brittany calls me by the nickname my late mother used. I left my list in the break room and invited the other employees to add their thoughts. To be fair I also made a list of things that I would *not* miss, like cleaning the bathrooms or various crabby things customers say. While writing that list was also therapeutic, I found it to be much shorter.

For two weeks now, some of my story time regulars have

visited me on what would have been our story time day. When I realized that story time was the number one thing I would miss, I found another location where I could offer it. Next week I again will be Miss Nina, the story time lady, and find myself surrounded by the bright and smiling faces of my little children.

As I move through these stressful stages of grief, I have found comfort in unexpected places and unexpected moments. The family that owns a nearby bakery brought us delicious baked treats several times. A local bagel store sent bagels and cream cheese. I found inspirational quotes about hardship and loss, and posted them by the time clock for all the employees to see. I read them every time I come to work. I told everyone about the little girl who organized the books and discovered she wasn't the only one—there were other customers seen organizing or sorting, and customers helping other customers find what they were searching for. Some of our customers are as much family as is our staff, and they are as sad as we are.

It's painful to go in to work, but I want to be there as much as I can. I want to remember what we had. So today I'm going to photograph my co-workers and put together something we can all keep, to remember what was so important to us for so long. I don't have her picture, but I hope I will always remember the little girl who reminded me that small miracles can sometimes happen when you need them most. Maybe she'll come back. But even if she doesn't, as I place the books she would read on that shelf, I'll think of her and smile.

~ Nina Schatzkamer Miller ~

A Little Fun
and Games

Work had gone beyond being a source of stress. In fact, it seemed to be nothing but stress. Everything connected to it also produced its own stress, and thinking about it when I was away from work piled even more stress onto that. I felt like I was being pressed from all sides.

I could tell I was irritable on the job. Usually my disposition is a sunny one, but the stress of trying to keep up with a flood of paperwork, trying to please my bosses, and worrying about the security and future of my job didn't lead to smiles. I was so wrapped up in the stress of trying to handle all of this that I found myself walking around in a fog most of the time, mumbling incoherent things to myself, miserable and feeling my hold on things slipping.

Home wasn't much better. The stress of work did not go away when I stepped through the front door. My wife smiled and hugged me, as encouraging and supportive as ever, and I'm ashamed to say I did little to justify her faith in me. I moped around a lot, lost in endless worries about work. I didn't feel like talking about the day or taking a walk or going to a movie or anything. What I really wanted to do was slide into bed, pull the covers over my head and tell everyone I was too sick to go to work.

But of course, that wasn't any kind of solution for my problems, or to the stress and pressure I was feeling. There had to be a way to handle all of this, to turn the negative feelings around and make things work better. I had to find an answer, and fast.

One day, I found myself swamped again. Dozens of people needed dozens of things, each at the same time. I had a report to present to my peers, and I knew I'd never be ready in time. So as I plowed into the paperwork, I gave half my attention to the work I needed for the meeting. I dashed off a page and literally slid it across my desk into the folder it needed to go into. It settled neatly into place.

I thought that was kind of cool, so the next time I had a page done I slid it across the desk, and watched in amazement as it slid perfectly in place on top of the first paper. This went on, with me sliding each page I completed, until I slid the very last one. I held my breath, and when it settled onto the top of the pile in the folder, I actually cheered. I closed the folder and let out a breath. I looked at the clock on my desk. I had finished both the report and the pile of paperwork with fifteen minutes to spare. I was ahead of the game.

It occurred to me that I had not felt any stress at all, caught up as I was in playing my made-up game. I'd done all the work I'd needed to do, but without the mountain of stress I'd normally feel. Could the fact that I was enjoying the game account for that?

I decided to find out. The rest of that week, whenever I had a particularly stressful assignment to tackle, I created a game or activity while I did it. When I was writing up my reports I made up songs about the various subjects and hummed them to myself. While I was processing an avalanche of files, I used color-coded folders and bet myself which color would end up making the highest stack. In short, I managed to fit some fun into the serious work I was doing.

After a week of such playful activity I began to stress about wasting time. Then I got to the end of the week and noticed that I had finished not a little of my work, not half of it, but all of the mind-numbing work that had been driving me crazy with stress. Adding a little harmless play had so freed me from the usual stress that haunted me that I could focus on the task at hand and get the job done. Not only that, but I began to notice that I was actually enjoying the work, something I hadn't felt in years.

So I continued to add a little fun to my workload. After a while my proficiency went up so much that my boss asked what was going on. I decided to come clean and tell him my secret. He stood and listened and frowned a lot, but he didn't say anything. However, later that afternoon he confided that he'd made anagrams out of the names of all the clients he'd talked to on the phone, had finished his business and had some genuine fun in the process.

So the fun continues, mixed in with a lot of serious work, and the stress that I thought I'd never be free of is a thing of the past. The thing I'd forgotten is that life is supposed to be filled with joy as much as drudgery. As long as I balanced the two, I got more done in a job that I was suddenly feeling very good about, all on account of a little fun and games.

~ John P. Buentello ~

Killer Jobs—
Stress and the
Workplace

Introduction

A stressful workplace may seem like the plague of the warp speed Information Age, but work and stress have walked hand in hand for eons. No doubt the workers who built the Egyptian pyramids grumbled about the long hours, unreasonable supervisors and nonexistent retirement plan.

By the twentieth century, employees began taking legal action to fight against all sorts of untenable working conditions. In 1934, a farm laborer sued his employer (and won) over the trauma he experienced when he happened upon a cow giving birth in a haystack. In 1960, a Michigan court awarded compensation to an auto assembly line worker who suffered a mental breakdown because he couldn't handle the speed and monotony of the assembly line.

It's unlikely you'll be stunned by an animal giving birth on your desk or driven to madness by someone standing over you with a stopwatch timing your every move. Even so, today's workforce seems to be a frazzled, stressed out bunch. Blame it on poor management, bad bosses, crazy-making co-workers or the relentless invasion of new technology—many of us view the workplace as a nerve-wracking minefield. According to the Bureau of Labor Statistics, one in every four of us sees our job as the main thing causing stress in our lives — even more so than money or family problems. Job pressures account for nearly seven in ten insurance stress claims. Stress can truly be considered a job hazard!

If your job is causing you to lose sleep or grind your teeth or any of the symptoms I've listed for you in "Signs of Workplace Stress" at the end of this chapter, get proactive about making changes. There are ways to effectively manage on-the-job stress. Read on and you'll see what I mean.

Communicate Well

A lot of workplace tension results from poor communication. Part of the problem is a disconnect between how well people think they communicate and how well they actually do. In a recent jobperformance.com analysis, 93 percent of managers said they answered employees' tough questions honestly. Some of them must be whispering — only 42 percent of employees believe the boss tells them the whole truth.

Another problem is the proliferation of communication choices. How many times have you e-mailed back and forth with a co-worker sitting three feet away from you? Facebook is replacing face-to-face interactions, often complicating matters and adding an impersonal layer of confusion into the mix, at least for those of us who favor actual conversations.

You can do your part to improve communication with

individual superiors and co-workers. Start by getting to know each person's communication style and preferences and then adjust accordingly. That doesn't mean becoming a therapist or twisting yourself into knots. It means learning to be a good listener and respecting individual differences.

You also have to develop thick skin. Don't take it personally if someone is abrupt and direct in their feedback style, but is then hypersensitive to those who return feedback in kind; it has nothing to do with you. Likewise, there are some people, especially those youthful digital natives, who truly prefer to get their information via e-mail or instant message rather than speaking words with their mouths; it may be helpful to learn their habits and their lingo, too.

Be consistent and attempt to address difficulties in communication before they fester into full-blown dramas that create tension for you and everyone else. My advice is to tackle tricky matters head on rather than circling around them. Be assertive yet compassionate. State your issues clearly, use specific examples, and do your best to keep it from getting too personal. It's a good idea to mentally rehearse conversations beforehand with the goal of eliminating unpleasant emotions and avoiding arguments. Situations may not always go the way you practiced, but at least you will have thought through some of the possibilities.

Many of the usual communication pitfalls can be eliminated by maintaining relationships that are polite and friendly, yet not too intimate, and that fit within the boundaries of your office's "corporate culture." Be mindful of this, whether you sit in the corner office, a cubicle, or telecommute, and when it comes to scenarios like work outings and holiday parties.

At all costs, avoid being lumped in with the whiners and gossips. If you've got a co-worker who frequently plops down next to your desk and proceeds to complain about everyone else in the office, smile, avoid commenting, and get back to work as soon as they take a breath. Don't go there with them or you risk guilt by association, which can lead to isolation from the mainstream office. Instead, cultivate support from as many sources as possible so there's always a lifeline when the seas get rough. (And you can be sure that if they're talking smack about the guy in accounting, they're probably trash talking you too.)

Instead, set an example like Nina Miller did when she worked at Borders during their bankruptcy liquidation. She posted inspirational notes near the time clock and supported her fellow employees in other ways. That's the way to face up to work adversity with dignity and class.

Are YOU the Problem?

You've probably come to realize there are all sorts of office personality clichés. There are the Whiners and the Gossips, who I've already mentioned. Then there are the Machiavellians, always scheming and plotting, as well as the Responsibility Dodgers, the Credit Hounds and the Micromanagers. The list goes on. The important question for you to ask yourself is, "Which type am I?" And then, "Am I the one who is creating stress in the office?"

This is a tough but important self-assessment. If you conclude you have unwittingly become the ground zero for office tension, it could be good news. Changing other people is hard. You have control over your own actions and words, so change is within *your* reach.

I've mentioned how helpful it is to understand the styles and preferences of others. It's just as useful to understand your own. For example, you may prefer to work independently rather than in a group, or you may wish to get your instructions up front and check in occasionally rather than continually. You might be able to mold your work environment to synch with your working style—if not, perhaps it's time to start thinking about finding a more suitable situation. But before you push the delete button, it's worth trying to express your wishes to your co-workers and bosses in a clear, nonjudgmental manner to see what can be done.

In any work scenario, your objective should be to cultivate a reputation as a team builder whether or not you are technically in charge. Team building is the art and science of allowing everyone to contribute their best skills and ideas without allowing anyone to overpower, micromanage or slack off.

Being a team-builder means developing the strong communication and listening skills we've already covered and by showing your commitment and excitement for the work. These traits are contagious and when there's a positive buzz in the air there's less room for negativity and dissension. It helps to make a point of recognizing the unique contributions each team member brings to the table and praising them in a sincere, meaningful manner.

Master this technique and not only will work be a happier place, you'll likely fast track your career.

Imagine Your Exit

Congratulations. You've been hired. Now it's time to plan your exit. Of course I'm not recommending immediately quitting as soon as you start a new job. I'm simply suggesting you define under what circumstances you *would* leave if you needed to. Do some thinking about the absolute values, morals and beliefs you'd never compromise no matter what. Know your personal line in the sand.

What would you do, for instance, if your boss asked you to lie about an earnings report to an investor? Or if she swore at you, using some pretty strong and explicit language in front of a group of co-workers? How about if someone you're sure does inferior work to your own is promoted ahead of you? What if you don't receive a raise within two years?

Deciding ahead of time what you won't tolerate helps you recognize "it" when "it" happens. Because your limits are clear it's less likely you'll be blindsided by circumstances that trip the wire on stress emotions such as anger, anxiety and fear. If a situation occurs that crosses your line, you won't experience that churn in your stomach for very long because you've already determined your course of action.

I recommend committing your exit plan to paper and reviewing it from time to time. So that you're always able to leave on your own terms, stay focused on cultivating professional relationships, keeping your résumé updated and staying sharp on technical skills — those should be givens anyway.

Also, draw a clear picture of what leaving will look like. We all know someone who told off the boss, threw his keys on the floor and stormed out. Satisfying in the moment, yes. But when you allow the flames of rage and resentment to flare up, you risk getting burned by the fumes, creating negative and stressful situations for yourself down the road. Remember: The boss you diss probably knows other potential bosses and can make your life miserable far beyond your tenure. So even if you've come to loathe your work situation, envision an exit that's polite and respectful, then stick with that vision should the time come.

Losing It

Unfortunately, sometimes it's not your choice to exit a job. We live in an age of "at will employment" where terminations and layoffs are part of the package. In terms of stress, losing your job ranks right up there on the Holmes and Rahe Stress Scale with marital troubles and the death of a close family member. Just the possibility of losing your job can fill you with dread. Just ask Nina Miller how it felt when her employer was going out of business.

If I can give you one piece of advice about work that you should take to heart, it's this: Don't let your job define you. Invest in what I like to call your "identity portfolio." This means always having things outside of work that help you feel fulfilled and engaged. Don't just be a shoe salesman. Be a shoe salesman who also paints and volunteers at the local food bank every Sunday.

People who take an extreme approach to their jobs by working crazy, long hours, neglecting their families or focusing on work to the exclusion of all else should examine their motives. If you're driven to live beyond your means or keep up with the Joneses or for some other superficial reason, I strongly urge you to pull back and consider nurturing other aspects of your life. If you've got a stressful job, follow John Buentello's lead and find a way to make it fun. This is a healthier approach to life that will save you from despair should you lose your job. Perhaps more importantly, a well-rounded identity provides outlets for blowing off steam while you're gainfully employed.

And if you do find yourself out of work, it's okay to mourn the loss of your job and allow yourself to feel depressed for a little while. This is normal and perhaps beneficial. However, don't allow the pity party to go on for too long. A resilient attitude is the key to bouncing back and finding a situation that's better than the one you had before. You might look upon a job loss as an opportunity to change careers, go back to school for more training, or look for a better situation. Instead of allowing yourself to be overcome with grief and angst, you can use unemployment as a chance to reenergize.

Signs of Workplace Stress

- Feeling anxious, irritable, or depressed
- Apathy, loss of interest in work
- Problems sleeping
- Fatigue
- Trouble concentrating
- Muscle tension or headaches
- Stomach problems
- Social withdrawal
- Loss of sex drive
- Using alcohol or drugs to cope

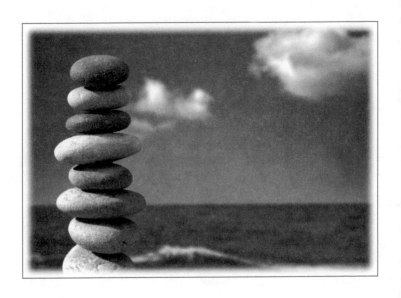

Chapter 4
Home Is Where the Heat Is

"Back" to Our Garden

When I left home for a ten-day silent yoga retreat, the last thing on my mind was my husband's chronic back pain. I know that doesn't sound very kind but I was more concerned about leaving my husband and children, my psychotherapy practice, and most importantly, the world of conversation, for ten days. But it was under the clear blue sky of the Arizona desert that suddenly without words I began to make sense of my husband's back pain.

Our retreat was taught by a beautiful and very gentle yoga teacher from Korea who led us through daily yoga poses and meditation practices that encouraged us to read our bodies like we would the novels by our bedsides. The aches and pains we felt in our backs, our shoulders, our knees, held our personal stories and were metaphors for our individual challenges. My chronic shoulder pain taught me about the burdens I carried, and as I learned more about myself, I thought more about my dear husband of close to thirty years.

He had always been active—an avid runner and tennis player. But in the last few years, he had suffered from low back pain that would often lead to evenings that we affectionately called the "hobbles." He loved gardening and his spring and summer blossoms were beautiful. But as his gardens flourished, my husband's weekends were filled to the brim with yard work. Often after a hot and sweaty afternoon, he'd pour a glass of water and comment, "Perhaps we could lay some more concrete, extend our porch—we really don't need so much grass and so many flowers!"

So as I moved through my yoga poses in silence and spent many hours in deep meditation, my reading of my husband's back pain became clear. The beauty of my husband's irises was taking on a darker hue. What began as a love and passion for Mother Earth was becoming more of a heavy weight and burden. I thought about how frequently the national news would report on homes collapsing due to tornados—individuals buried by the disaster. Suddenly I recognized that my husband and I were being buried by the demands of our home and our work, suffering from our own psychological tornado.

Even though most of our days were spent in silence on my retreat, infrequent check-ins with our families were allowed. Cell phone service wasn't always the best so the important conversation I needed to have with my husband wasn't so easy.

"What, lovey, I'm losing you, can't hear you..." I heard my husband say through static.

But finally it all became clear. "We should think about moving, simplifying our lives, working less!" I said with great emphasis.

My husband rationally answered, "But why?"

I explained that his back pain had to be related to the pressure he put on himself to make our home and yard look beautiful and how sad it would be to spend our next fifty years being driven by our responsibilities. It was the combination of both the physical and psychological strain that landed him in the "hobbles." I wanted him to stop turning his "back" on himself and his wellbeing. Our life was our garden; it was time we weeded out those aspects that were bringing him so much pain. Obviously, our brief conversation was just the beginning but I knew I was laying the groundwork for something wonderful that felt so much more hopeful than laying concrete.

I returned from my week of silence with a few short words on my to-do list. "Simplify," "Move," and find time to "Breathe." And now, five years later, we live a block away from our larger house, in a small home with a beautiful little garden. The flowers are blossoming as I write this. My husband and I have both shed the burden of working too many hours. His infrequent low back pain is just a reminder he's pushing too hard both physically and psychologically. We find time to take better care of ourselves, infusing yoga into our daily lives where we stretch ourselves toward a sense of peace instead of pain.

— Priscilla Dann-Courtney —

The Sweet Stuff

I stood beside the snack table that displayed the various holiday treats for my daughter's pre-kindergarten class. Cupcakes with thick frosting, cookies with colorful sprinkles, cakes of every shape and flavor. Balancing my two-year-old son on my hip, I added my bottle of apple juice to the array of items. Suddenly, I felt inadequate. Was I a bad mom for bringing the apple juice instead of baking? I promised myself, the next party, I would be like the other proud moms who stood closely beside their baked items as if to say, "See me? I baked. I'm a good mom."

The next party came before I knew it. As a working mom, I tried my best to squeeze in everything—quality time, play time, laundry, grocery shopping, cleaning, cooking—with work. Now I added cookies. I managed to bake some from a mix and brought them in proudly. I placed them on the table among the other baked goods. Immediately, someone turned to me. "Oh, cookies. Are they homemade?" It was then, I realized, there was a rating on the bake scale. From a box, low score. From a mix, just passing. From scratch... now that's topnotch. The same rule applied for church functions as well as large family gatherings.

Trying to keep up with the other moms with my family and my schedule was added stress I didn't need.

"Could you bring the cookies?"

I'd be baking at midnight.

"Could you bring potato salad?"

I'd be peeling those potatoes for hours.

For years I added more and more to my plate, excuse the pun. One Sunday morning, while preparing my meal for an after-church dinner, I found myself running behind. My daughter couldn't find her school shoes and her dress shoes were too tight. Now an unexpected run to the store was needed to avoid the embarrassment of wearing dirty sneakers with a dress. My mind raced. Would we be late? Would the food stay warm? Would it taste bad if it had to be reheated? I grumbled all the way, sighing as we hastily tried on shoes and raced to the checkout.

Eventually arriving at church, I smiled and handed my well-made dinner to the ladies in the kitchen. Then I glanced at my daughter, standing there quietly, teary-eyed with shiny shoes. What was I doing? I realized my homemade dinner was not worth what I gave up to make it. It was then I decided to de-stress my obligations.

The following week I received a phone call. "We're having a family picnic tomorrow. I forgot to call in advance. You are down for macaroni or potato salad."

I glanced at the clock: 6:30 p.m. Right then, my kids called from the other room where they were sitting, popcorn in hand.

"Mommy... the movie's coming on!"

I hung up the phone, snuggled next to my kids and grabbed a handful of popcorn.

The next day, the kids and I took our time as we got ready for the picnic. I helped them find their shoes, and I braided my daughter's hair. We sang silly songs in the car. On the way, I detoured and swung into the grocery store. I quickly bought two pounds of macaroni salad from their fantastic deli, dumped it into my yellow bowl, sprinkled it with paprika and covered it with plastic wrap. Done. We continued on, singing all the way.

I have continued this easy, no-stress way of cooking for every event since. Pre-made cupcakes from Sam's Club. Holiday pies from a bakery. It freed up my time, was stress-free, delicious and easy! Baking with the kids was fun and done more often due to the miracle of tub cookies, slice and bake, and pre-sliced in a tray. My kids loved how easily we baked and how good those warm cookies tasted.

My kids are now in college. They can recall childhood things such as movie nights, silly songs, and games at the fair. But honestly, they can't remember one cupcake or cookie from a school party.

Today my son called from his apartment. We only talked briefly before he announced, "I have to go now Mom. I'm baking."

"Really?" I asked, rather surprised, but happy. "What are you baking?"

"Cookies."

I smiled. I was a good mom.

~ Judy A. Weist ~

Bite by Bite

"Mom, I can't do this." My teenage son Bret stood in front of me with his hands outstretched, full of papers.

"Can't do what?" I half-looked at him while preparing supper.

"All this!" He waved his hands up and down to show me. "There's no way I can do everything my teachers are asking me to do!"

I stopped what I was doing and turned to face him. I had never seen him so upset. He was my jovial, carefree son. He made good grades in school and nothing ever seemed to bother him. As I studied his face, I could see tears brimming in his eyes accompanying the look of panic.

Walking over to the kitchen table, I sat down and motioned him to join me.

"Show me what you have to do."

Bret plopped down in a chair and dropped the papers in a stack in front of him.

"Ms. Jones, my chemistry teacher, wants me to make a project for the Science Fair."

"Okay. And what else?"

"I have an algebra test next week that will be one-third of our semester grade!"

I knew how Bret hated algebra, which always gave him trouble.

"And I have to write an essay for English composition. And midterms are the next week! I need to study for them and I have to get help with Spanish. There's no way I can do everything!"

His hands shook as he picked up each assignment. It broke my heart to see him so stressed out. I wanted to help him, yet I couldn't do the work for him. I could relate to his dilemma though.

In my job as a sales manager, there had been many stressful times. Caught in the middle, I had to please upper management by producing results from my sales team as well as deal with ten individuals who each had concerns with making their quotas, taking care of their customers and personal issues.

I was particularly stressed out when I had to plan a sales meeting for the company. At that time, I was in charge of the agenda, setting up the presentations, arranging the people who would participate, ordering supplies, and so on. My performance was on the line and under the closest scrutiny at these times.

As much as I wanted to run away and hide from the responsibility, I knew I had to handle it. And even though I had my doubts about the outcome, I wanted things to run well. How did I handle it and not implode? I made a list. I listed everything that had to be done, then I put a deadline on each item and organized the list according to what had to be done first, second, and so on.

Back in the kitchen, I looked at Bret and said, "You don't have to do everything at once. You can do one at a time. Let's make a list of what you need to do."

So, one by one, we listed each item. Then we put the due date next to the item. Next we separated the items into parts; for instance, the chemistry project needed supplies. So we put a deadline on getting the supplies. He had a friend who could help him with Spanish, so we had to factor that time in. As we worked on prioritizing the tasks, I saw my son visibly relax.

When we finished with the list, I asked, "Do you think you can do this now?"

He smiled and I saw his confidence return. "Sure! Thanks, Mom!"

From that day on, Bret made lists for everything he had to do. I had to laugh when I saw lists on pieces of paper lying around, but I knew the process worked for him, as it did for me. Bret completed all his assignments and kept his good grades.

There's an adage that asks, "How do you eat an elephant?" The answer is, "One bite at a time."

— Marilyn Turk —

Just Breathe

"Have you seen the wedding list?" I asked my husband.

"Nope... haven't seen it," Mark answered.

As I shuffled through the stack of papers on the kitchen table, my elbow brushed against the "Have a Nice Day" mug, spilling the creamy mocha concoction onto the newly cleaned carpet. Too paralyzed to breathe, I felt a tear trickle down my cheek, followed by another and another, until they fell beneath my hands onto the pile of bills and receipts.

It was too much! Our son was getting married in three weeks; we had out-of-town guests who needed a place to stay; and we were selling our house, and packing up thirty-five years of marriage in preparation for a move to Cuenca, Ecuador—our retirement destination!

While I sat with my head in my hands, the phone rang beside me. "Yeah, what do you want?" I answered, without thinking.

"It's Kathy—your best friend—remember me?" came the reply. "Are you okay? You sound like you're having a crummy day."

It had been weeks since I heard the voice of my dear friend and I could tell she was genuinely concerned.

Kathy and I hadn't connected in weeks and she was calling to cheer me up.

"I'm sorry, but it's just so overwhelming," I blubbered. "There's so much to do and not enough time!" As I shared my fears about our house not selling, out-of-town guests arriving with no place to stay, and a house littered with boxes for an overseas move, I heard Kathy exhale a sigh.

"Whoa, girl... you need to take a deep breath!" she said. "Would you like to meet for lunch? I have time this week. I can even meet you halfway."

Before I had a chance to respond, Kathy reminded me to practice breathing. "Hee-hee-huu... shallow breaths and blow," she prompted. "I'm a Lamaze instructor—remember?"

"How could I forget?" I blurted into the phone. "But I'm not having a baby!"

"No, but you're losing one," Kathy replied softly.

A lump formed in my throat when I realized that not only were we moving to another continent, but our baby was getting married. As soon as I placed the phone in its cradle, I realized that breathing is how I made it through labor. It helped me focus on something other than the pain. And just maybe it could help with a wedding and a move!

Hee-hee-huu, I practiced. "Breathe in energy... exhale stress," I told myself. "Shallow breaths and blow!"

Over the next couple of days, I practiced breathing while I packed up boxes, prepared for a wedding shower, and "labored" through thirty-five years of memories. Night after night, I stayed up until 3:00 a.m., scanning important documents, family photos, and memorabilia, but I didn't feel stressed. The breathing exercises were working!

I started to feel slightly better on the third day when I could actually breathe in deeply without clutching my chest for more air. The wedding plans were going smoothly and we finally had an offer on our home that we could both live with. It looked like we were going to have a wedding and a move to Ecuador after all. As I started to take in a cleansing breath, the phone rang.

"I have good news and bad news," announced the realtor. "The new owners want to move in and settle over the Memorial Day weekend!"

"They want what?" I protested. "I mean they can't. That's the wedding weekend!" I shouted into the phone. "I have guests coming from California and they need a place to stay. It's simply not going to work out."

Our realtor stood firm. "The new owners need to settle by the end of the month and it's in your best interest to do so," she said.

After the phone call, I knew what to do. Hee-hee-huu, I practiced. "Breathe in energy... exhale stress," I told myself. "Shallow breaths and blow!"

Over the next several weeks, I had more opportunities to practice my Lamaze, including when I found out the box labeled "wedding" accidently got sent to the incinerator instead of the church. But all was forgiven when the bride and groom danced up the aisle for the first time as husband and wife. When it came time for the mother-groom dance—I breathed through that too, making sure I didn't hyperventilate during the four minutes and thirty seconds of our song. The wedding was a success and so was the move.

It's been over a year since the kids said "I do" and we arrived at our retirement destination in Ecuador, the land of "eternal springtime" and *siempre mañana* (always tomorrow). I rarely have to use my Lamaze breathing anymore, except for the other day when a *taxista* (taxi driver) slammed on his brakes for a pack of llamas crossing the street. As we slid into the intersection, my husband grabbed my arm and whispered in my ear, "Just breathe!"

~ Connie K. Pombo ~

Home
Is Where
the Heat Is

Introduction

Your home is your sanctuary. It's your castle, your personal safe haven. And the beautiful family that resides with you? They're the most treasured people in your life. Yet even the happiest of homes can still be the epicenter of stress.

While home and loved ones are usually a source of joy, they can also be a big source of tension and stress. Kids, partners, siblings and parents place demands on you. Conflicts arise. Things break. Bills and laundry pile up. Sometimes it's enough to make your head explode! And that's even before you toss a doozie like divorce, a new baby or surly teenagers into the mix.

Just how much is home life stressing out the average American? The American Psychological Association's most recent Stress in America survey found that more than half of all Americans lie awake at night worrying about family-related issues and over 70 percent of parents cite family responsibilities as a significant source of stress. Divorce ranks just below death of a loved one on most stress scales. With about 50 percent of Americans admitting they have anxiety about paying the rent or mortgage, even the literal roof over our heads is giving us agita.

For sure, home life strife is complicated by a tangle of emotions—everything from love to sadness to pride to anger to exhaustion. That doesn't mean you can't get a handle on it though. Learning to cope strengthens familial bonds and prepares you to deal with the larger crises that inevitably crop up. As the stories in this chapter demonstrate so nicely, once you strike the right balance, peace and harmony can prevail within the four walls of your home, so that both you and your family are happier and healthier. I've got some sensible advice for you on how to do just that.

A Lifetime Commitment

It sounds like it should be the most natural thing in the world: Have a conversation with a family member that involves reasonable dialog and mutual understanding. If only it were always that simple.

No one gets under your skin quite like someone who is related to you by DNA or marriage. Maybe it's because we feel so comfortable in our relationships or they are so enmeshed that deep down we don't think a little shouting (or the silent treatment) can cause any long-term harm.

Think again. What you say and how you say it to a family member matters a lot because they're the people with whom you have the most at stake. This is doubly true when there are children in the mix. Your overall communication style impacts them on multiple levels—something to keep in mind at all times but especially when adults in the household aren't getting along.

Studies show that kids whose parents engage in a war of finger pointing and blame often have lower math and social skills than children from stable homes.

Whether you're going through a nasty divorce, you're at war with another family member, or acrimony is merely par for the course in your household, you owe it to your children to dial it down. It's your lifetime responsibility to ensure the effects of negative energy don't spill over onto your child. That means co-parenting with mutual respect, setting up civil rules of engagement everyone can live with and resisting the temptation to use your offspring as spies or go betweens. Do it for the sake of your children but don't be surprised if it helps make things better for you too.

Assess the Situation

Let me share something I tell my patients that's often difficult for them to hear: One of the best ways to improve family dynamics is by taking a long hard look at yourself. You may be so sure that everyone else is wrong or that they need to be taught a lesson, you don't realize that you yourself are causing problems. Are you fanning the flames, taking the bait or falling into any of the other common traps of poor relationship management? The strong emotions created by weak communication can take on a life of their own. You can become so preoccupied with being right or winning an argument, that you don't realize it's more productive to let go of something that is ultimately insignificant.

I know that taking a personal inventory can be particularly

challenging. It's tough to admit that you are the one who needs to change your ways. Trust me, it's always worth it. Far from giving in, it's a way of stepping back and allowing yourself to gain control of your thoughts, feelings and behavior.

Actually, if there's a lot of turmoil in your house and misunderstandings swarm like bees, it's not a bad idea for every single family member to engage in some self-reflection. I'm not saying it's easy to ask them to do this—it's hard enough getting everyone to clear their own dishes off the table—but if you take the lead perhaps they'll follow your example. If not, you're still ahead of the game because at least you've taken responsibility for your own actions.

Strike a Balance

Good communication can go a long way towards depressurizing home life. Try zipping your lip and using your ears once in a while. You'll be amazed at how much loved ones are dying for someone to listen more and judge less. So rather than offering unsolicited advice to your angsty sixteen-year-old (who won't appreciate hearing your opinion anyway) let him tell his side of the story for a change. You don't have to agree. You just have to listen.

Pick your spots. It's okay to speak your mind with firm composure and let your loved ones know what you need when the situation calls for it. You may think your wishes are obvious to everyone, but they aren't always. Articulating them directly without accusations can be an amazingly effective way to defuse tense situations.

Putting differences aside and giving family members the respect and consideration they crave helps when there are big issues to resolve. It helps in handling the small, everyday issues too. In my house, for instance, I try to tell my wife where I'm going every time I leave the room, even if I'm just going to the kitchen for a drink. This may seem like over sharing but it helps improve our communication and avoid misunderstandings.

Find Support

Whether you've asked for it or not, never feel guilty about accepting help when you really need it. Welcome it gratefully and graciously wherever it comes from — and it can often come from unexpected places. When one of my patient's husbands unexpectedly had a stroke, the parents at her child's school got together and organized a support system for her. People she'd never spoken to stopped by with a week's worth of meals. Someone offered her rides to and from the hospital. Another mom organized play dates for her child every day after school. She described it as an incredibly touching experience; it opened her eyes to how willing people are to help someone in need — a good life lesson.

Also, if things are really rough at home, I urge you to talk it out with someone. I'm not saying you should constantly whine about your troubles, but keeping your frustrations bottled up does neither you nor anyone else any good. Sharing lifts burdens, both great and small, off your shoulders.

If you don't have a sympathetic, trusted confidante, see a

therapist. Actually, consider therapy even if you are blessed with a strong support system. A trained professional can often provide a fresh perspective and insights into your family issues. She can act as a mediator to defuse family tensions and help resolve age old grudges. Your therapist has no bone to pick with anyone so she's free to act as the neutral party who offers fair and honest advice. Plus you should never worry about a therapist gossiping about your business to the neighbors. She's honor bound to keep your secrets safe. When merited, urge other family members to seek professional counseling and consider family counseling as well.

Prepare Yourself

Sometimes you can see problems coming from a mile away—and sometimes they hit you like a bus. Preparing yourself to weather stormy situations isn't always possible but there are times when it is.

Take having a baby, a great example of a very "happy" form of stress. The birth of a child is one of the most joyous events in a person's life. However, along with all the joy comes 2:00 a.m. feedings, colic and a charming little phenomenon known as dirty diapers. You can't stop these inevitabilities from coming but you can minimize the stress they cause. Get as much rest as you can between feedings, set up a schedule to distribute the work and get as much as possible done before the baby arrives. While you're at it, set up a visiting schedule so you aren't bombarded with a well-meaning crowd on the baby's first day home.

(There's always that clueless aunt who asks the new mother to brew some coffee for her.) When you do have visitors, don't be shy about referring them to the handwritten list of things they can do to help or asking them to cover for you while you catch a nap.

The fact is with a little forethought there are probably plenty of home life issues you can prepare yourself for, or at least certain aspects of them. That's the idea behind working mom Judy Weist's lists. She realized that she became overwhelmed unless she got organized. Instead of passing the pressure on to the rest of her household she passed the gift of organization down to her stressed-out son. That's a nice outcome.

On a larger scale, you can put a little money aside for a rainy day to help fix a leaky roof. Learn everything you can about caring for an elderly parent to avoid making mistakes and maintain your sanity. You can't expect the unexpected but you can expect that something unexpected is inevitable.

Make Time

Just as flowers need water and sunshine to thrive, so do relationships benefit from careful cultivation. Setting aside time for your loved ones is essential for staying close and connected. It could be that your young daughter is acting up because she doesn't know how to express her desire to spend more time with you. Perhaps that's why your spouse is acting up for that matter! Maybe it's time to consider a smaller house like Priscilla Dann-Courtney did.

Without being too morbid, I like to remind my patients about the information that is going to appear on their gravestones. I've often heard that the "dash" that separates their birth date and death date represents their life. I ask them—and I'll ask you—what will your dash represent: All the hours you put in at work or the fact that you were a great dad, an attentive mother, a caring son or a loving wife?

This not so subtle reminder about the importance of prioritizing family is something we all can use from time to time. We can get wrapped up in work and everyday minutia but we shouldn't forget the goodbye kisses, the small thoughtful gestures and the "I love yous." Though their annoying habits can drive you up the wall and they can be so frustrating they bring you to tears, your family is your one and only. Home is truly where the heat is. Take that to heart.

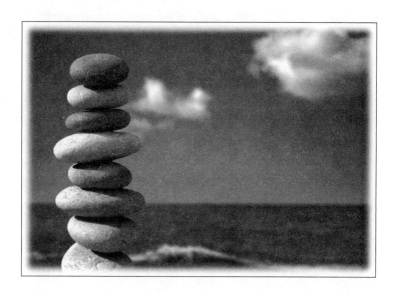

Chapter 5
Preventing Monetary Meltdown

Tick Tock

11:25 P.M. Sleep doesn't come readily these nights. Quite a conundrum considering that the days go by without any rest or downtime. By the time I haul my body up the two flights of stairs to our bedroom, I hunger for sleep. I brush my teeth with the energy of a slug. (Thank goodness for electric toothbrushes.) The anticipation of a deep slumber is the only thing keeping me vertical. I literally crawl into bed as my husband, John, is already there lying in the dark. His gentle snoring guides me to my side of the bed. I am there, horizontal, smiling at the sheer thought of motionless sleep. My eyes close.

11:35 p.m. Eyes wide open, my body tenses as I listen to John's not-so-gentle snoring. My thoughts begin to race. I am all consumed by the minutia of everyday chores. At the same time, I am wondering why no one has called me back regarding employment. Over the past two years, I have sent résumés that now lie in a stack two inches deep on my desk. Who knows how many ads I have answered? I lost track last year when I realized that counting unacknowledged résumés was counterproductive, definitely not an inspirational way to spend my time. Maybe I should count them at night, instead of sheep. One to a museum in Brooklyn, two, to a nonprofit film school in New York, three, to an adult daycare center in Rye.... No such luck. Still awake.

12:40 a.m. I am thinking about the money we saved to buy a second home that would serve as a college fund for our two children. Over the years we congratulated ourselves on how clever we were, having the house on Long Island that forced us to save for college, and a home in Connecticut as our retirement fund. We had a nice stock portfolio. We were set. We often commented that in our shared security, the only way we could lose would be for the entire country's financial status to crash.

1:15 a.m. I'm thinking about the bills on the table and those yet to arrive. I think about the color red that, for the first time, finds a place in my checkbook as I try to balance it daily. I'm worried about John's health. Since the company he worked for closed, he has been working hard trying to recreate himself through his own company. Starting his own business has affected his health, inducing sleep apnea and heartburn. I worry about the substantial health insurance bill hovering at the top of my bills-to-pay pile. The bill that more than doubled when we were forced to find our own insurance. I listen carefully to John's interrupted breathing.

1:40 a.m. I sit up, letting the night breeze cool off my sweaty body as hot flashes run up and down, making me a little nauseous. This is heightened by the realization that my son's college tuition is due at the end of the month. With John self-employed and me still looking, we don't have the luxury of a regular paycheck. Despite my frugality, we haven't been able to keep up with the monthly bills that continually invade our mailbox, let alone rebuild the six-month emergency fund we lost to the present economy. I feel my heart race trying to keep up with the continual hot flashes and John's deafening snore.

2:15 a.m. I'm thinking about the latest job I applied for, wondering if maybe I should call and make sure they got my application. It is quite disheartening, to say the least, to not even get a call or an interview. I would like to think I am overqualified as opposed to saying it's my age, but I feel my age has disqualified me from the final picks. My mother always said that once you turn fifty, you are less marketable. I never wanted to believe her, but it could be true. I love working, learning something new, meeting new people and realizing I'm not a stupid, tired woman. Well, maybe tired.

3:00 a.m. My mental list begins to grow for tomorrow's (today's) domestic needs. Since I'm not bringing in money and the kids are out of the house, I need to make sure I'm doing enough to justify myself. Sick. All this self-imposed pressure. I think about our now dwindling 401K and how I had happily contributed to it in the past.

3:28 a.m. I am thinking back to when John and I were young. Newly engaged and looking to be married at a local church. It was a tiny white church beside the water on Long Island, down the street from my parents' home. When we met the pastor, we were thrilled to find a young woman, Cynthia, who literally greeted us with open arms. We introduced ourselves, telling her how we met, where we worked and lived. After our romantic reviews, Cynthia looked at us and asked, "Which one of you will be handling the checkbook?" I was taken aback. In preparation for our meeting, I had reviewed an old Sunday school class curriculum, expecting questions about religion and faith. Financial questions were not on my agenda.

John looked at me. I looked at John. With no credit cards and barely a hundred dollars between the both of us, I said, "We'll share it. We plan on sharing everything." I was very young! Cynthia closed her notebook and said, "Come back next week when you have talked it over and have an answer." We looked baffled as she told us that in the course of a marriage, when money gets tight, finances will be the main thing that will test your relationship.

She was right. For over twenty years, I have done the bills and when money gets tight, I hold that information close to the vest. Being the major breadwinner, I feel John doesn't need the additional pressure of my accounting results.

3:35 a.m. I look over at John. No snoring. I get close to his face, listening for breathing as I had often done with my sleeping infants. He opens his eyes and says, "Something you want to talk about?"

"Just thinking," I say.

"I noticed. You've been rolling around like a billiard ball all night. What's up?"

Still half asleep, I bombard John with it all. The bills. The resentment I feel at not having a job. My domestic inadequacies. For good measure, I even throw in that I miss the kids off at college.

"Wow," he says, "been holding all that in long?" With that he hugs me. "Everything will sort itself out as soon as my clients start paying. We both have to be better at discussing our financial status. It's been eating at me too. The money is coming in, just not on a regular basis, so we need to talk more often, perhaps a weekly dinner meeting?" he says with a smile in his voice.

"As far as a job for you, the world is stupid for not hiring you. Before you know it you will find something you will love, so enjoy time home while you can. Maybe visit the kids. You know, if we ever feel like our financial nut is too great, we can sell the houses and find a small apartment. Does it really matter where we live?"

After more than twenty years together, it most certainly does not. We were in it together, wherever. I lie down in his arms and before I know it...

6:15 a.m. I hear the stirring of our eight-year-old mastiff, Max, as he advises me it's time to wake up and tend to his needs. I go downstairs to be greeted by a limping 125-pound sweetie in need of an ACL surgery and instead of worrying about how we will pay for the procedure, I think about how much I love our time together.

6:30 a.m. I put on my jacket and we slip outside for an early morning walk. The sun rises slowly, quietly, brightly. Upon our return, the local paper has found its way onto the driveway. I pick it up and go inside. I feed Max, make some coffee and open the paper to the classifieds. Maybe this will be the night I finally get some sleep.

~ Anna Koopman ~

All You Can Do

"I'm sorry," I explained to the debt collector on the phone, "that's all the money I can send right now. I will pay more when I can." I listened to her lecture on the importance of meeting my obligations, something I had endured every week or so since the car accident that had left me unable to work full-time, then hung up and dissolved into tears.

Three months earlier I had been stopped in traffic when a young woman drove into the back of my car and pushed me into the SUV in front of me. The back of my seat broke. As I fell backward, my pelvis hit the steering wheel, my knee hit the steering column with such force that it broke the column, and my shins were cut in several places. She had been driving about 40 mph and tearfully admitted that she was distracted and never put her foot on the brake pedal. To everyone's astonishment I had no broken bones, but suffered two badly sprained ankles, a very swollen knee, some spinal injuries and a concussion that left my mind cloudy for a few weeks.

My car was badly damaged. The engine had been pushed in toward the cab from the force of hitting the vehicle in front of me, and the back of the car had been pushed toward the cab from the impact. Seeing the car afterward, it was hard to believe I wasn't much more badly injured. Many months later I joked about being the meat in a car sandwich.

Self-employed in a job that required physical strength and being on my feet, I was unable to work for a while, and later could only work limited hours. As a single mother working to put a child through college, I had long ago canceled my disability insurance because the premiums were too high. I knew that at some point I would get a financial settlement, but that didn't help my current situation. With my limited income I still had to pay my business expenses, my rent and other home-related expenses, tuition, and my credit card bill. I was paying out far more than I was taking in, and my savings quickly evaporated. The physical pain I had was greatly overshadowed by the emotional stress of trying to stay on top of my obligations. I had cut household expenses to the bone, and still I was unable to make the minimum payment on the credit card bill.

For months I struggled financially, the stress of it slowing down my physical recovery. At times my body would seize in spasms, but the tears that fell came more from worry than pain. My mind was filled with fear. My blood pressure had risen dangerously. What if I never fully recovered? How would I earn a living? I was plagued with doubt, and terrified that I would no longer be able to pay my daughter's college tuition.

Then I received more devastating news. My older sister had been diagnosed with terminal cancer and did not have long to live. My spirit was crushed. In anguish I asked God how I could bear this on top of everything else. And then he asked me a question: "Have you done your best?" I pondered that for a moment, unsure what he was asking. I was working as much as I could. I was spending as little as possible. I was keeping up with my physical therapy. I could do nothing to save my sister. Yes, as far as I knew I had done my best. "Then that is all you can do. Now stand and wait."

The question had caught me off guard. My answer and the response offered no real solution, but peace floated down on me and lifted my spirit. Within moments the phone rang; the credit card debt collector was calling again. They called once or twice a week, asking the same questions, getting the same answer, then giving the same lecture. But instead of holding my breath and dreading the conversation, when she asked again when I could get current with the minimum payment, my answer was somewhat different.

"I'm sorry, but there is no change in my circumstances. I'm not sure when I can get current. I know you are just doing your job, but I can't do anything more than what I am doing and the stress has been affecting my physical wellbeing. I'm not trying to be evasive. As soon as I can I will get current. In the meantime, I just can't let this ruin my health. I'm not willing to have a heart attack wondering when I can pay you."

There was silence for a while. Then I heard her speak in a quiet voice, "Good for you. It's not worth dying for. Of course, I'm still going to have to keep making these calls." I thanked her and hung up, then took the deepest breath I had in months.

My life did not become instantly easier. My sister passed away about twelve weeks after her diagnosis, and I still miss her every day despite the years that have passed. Over time I recovered as much as I ever will. I have some chronic pain, but overall my life is very good. I am still self-employed, although the economy has made things tight once more. But since that day, whenever things go sideways, I take a moment and ask myself, "Am I doing the best I can?" If the answer is no, I make necessary changes. If the answer is yes, then I stand and wait. It has never failed to relieve my stress, never failed to give me strength. It works for small inconveniences as well as bigger issues. Do your best—that is all that can be asked of you.

~ Beth Arvin ~

Preventing
Monetary
Meltdown

Introduction

Almost everyone has conflicted feelings about money. Does it buy happiness or is it the root of all evil? Believe it or not, this conundrum is the subject of some intense scientific scrutiny.

Recently, Princeton University researchers came down on the side of the argument that says money can buy happiness — up to a point. By surveying the earnings and attitudes of nearly half a million Americans, they were able to link an increase in a person's day-to-day contentment with their income until it hit $75,000 per year. People with smaller paychecks expressed the least amount of everyday satisfaction but once their earnings rose above the $75,000 threshold, daily happiness didn't blossom any further. More zeros in the bank account did correlate with a greater overall sense of success, just not with a larger daily dose of joy.

On the flip side of the coin (yes, pun intended) having mere thoughts about money seems to leave us feeling more hardhearted towards our fellow man. In experiments where people were reminded of the all mighty dollar in conversation or after viewing monetary images on a computer screensaver, they spent less time helping others, sat farther away from other people and preferred solitary pursuits. Other studies reported that when people make a lot of money, they spend a higher percentage of income on themselves rather than charity or on others. While no one would consider this evil behavior, it's far from kind, loving and generous.

Money Puts the "S" in $tress

This sort of research doesn't really help resolve anything about our complicated relationship with finances. Everyone knows money can be one of the most stressful aspects of our lives whether we have a lot or a little. The most recent American Psychological Association's Stress In America poll found more than 75 percent of Americans worry about money for one reason or another; about 70 percent say it's their number one source of worry. In another survey by *Parade Magazine*, money was cited as the leading cause of conflict in marriages. Still another analysis, this time by Financial Finesse Reports, estimated 60 percent of illness is directly or indirectly caused by financial stress, with middle aged, middle income women (those who make between $60,000 and $74,000) feeling financial pressures the most intensely.

I think money is such a stressful, even painful topic for many people because it's shrouded with uncertainty and in many instances it's simply taboo. We fear and revere money yet understand almost nothing about it. Consequently, a lot of us are appallingly bad financial managers. In all fairness, we weren't taught to balance our checkbooks when we learned how to read, nor were we required to take money management courses in high school or college, so the majority of us reach adulthood with little instruction on how to handle our paychecks. I think this is why the pastor was wise to ask Anna Koopman who would handle the checkbook. It's a question few couples consider before they get married.

This fact is unfortunate because evidence shows a clear link between poor money management skills and financial stress, with a very direct correlation between the degree of financial stress someone faces and their ability to manage their expenses, control their debt, and pay their bills on time. I know plenty of people all up and down the ladder of financial success who don't follow a budget, do little in the way of financial planning, and don't do any serious financial preparation for the unexpected. Even those who say they're pretty mellow about their financial future may not feel the same later in life, since more than half admit they haven't put much effort into saving for retirement or protecting their assets.

What's Your Money Personality?

Combined with lack of training, I also believe your "money personality" plays a strong role in your emotional reaction and conduct towards money. The feelings and behaviors you have toward dollars and cents, which may have formed as early as childhood, can govern your spending, giving, and investment decisions. Understanding these powerful forces can help you conquer financial fears and perhaps help curb some undesirable financial behaviors too. Let's do a quick review of these money personalities. See if you can spot yours in the mix:

Show Off: For you, money equals prestige. You spend it for recognition and whether you realize it or not, you spread cash around to pump up your self-esteem. Your monetary strategy revolves around keeping up with the Joneses even if you can't afford to.

High Roller: You take risks even when the stakes are high and even if there's a chance you won't be able to cover potential losses. You save nothing for a rainy day, thinking you'll figure something out when the time comes. If you don't watch it, your tendency towards reckless spending gets you into trouble.

Ostrich: Money scares you so much you feel it's best to stick your head in the sand and not think about it too much. You hope for the best but fear the worst. Your approach towards money is rooted in dread and ignorance. You likely fear what you don't know and will never take a risk.

Squirrel: You're a saver and some might even say a penny pincher. You shop on sale and don't feel the need to have the nicest car or the fanciest home. Careful planning is your financial hallmark. However, sometimes you're so vigilant you deprive yourself of affordable luxuries that make life pleasurable.

Beginner: Whether you're newly divorced, fresh out of college or you're otherwise striking out on your own for the first time, you've never had to handle your own finances before. You have no clue whatsoever how to manage your money. You learn by trial and error and of course your expensive financial education comes from the school of hard knocks.

I certainly don't claim to be a financial management expert. However, my job as a psychologist is to help my patients gain some perspective about their money-related stressors. All of the personalities I just described are susceptible to worries about money. I like to emphasize the importance of exploring these feelings and attitudes, not necessarily with the goal of changing your personality type but as a way to make peace with money.

Tips for All Types

Do you know how much money is in your various bank accounts, the exact amount of your monthly car payment and your total monthly food budget? Few people do. Ostriches and Beginners may not because they can't bear to know the answers. Show Offs and High Rollers might figure it doesn't matter because they'll continue to spend no matter what. Squirrels are the most likely to check their balances and budgets regularly, though I've known plenty of people within this money personality category who sock away dollars while remaining clueless about the state of their financial health. As tough as it can be to face up to facts, I think one of the most effective ways to defuse money stress is by learning all you can about where you are and where you need to be. Ostriches, for example, may discover their finances aren't as bad as they feared. Or if their situation isn't where it needs to be, as was the case with Beth Arvin, at least they can come up with a plan to improve their situation and "do the best they can." For High Rollers and Show Offs, a thorough financial audit can be a wakeup call to curb high stakes behavior. Learning to manage the rush that comes with spending and luxury is also worth the time investment. Really, no matter how you feel about money, knowledge is power—and an incredibly effective stress reducer.

Again, I'm not a financial planner so I can't give you step-by-step instructions on how to balance the books or tell you what the makeup of your stock portfolio should be. I can however emphasize the importance of knowing as much as possible about your finances. There are plenty of ways to get there: Hire a money manager, buy a financial software package, read a book, take a class, ask a money savvy friend for help. Put your qualms aside and dive in.

If at all possible, enlist your partner in the audit and budgeting process. If he or she won't or can't participate, forge ahead anyway. Although it's ideal if you and your partner match up in terms of personalities and objectives, I often see couples who can't get together on this. I urge you not to let a reluctant partner stop you from getting a handle on your money. The idea is to alleviate your stress, whether it's shared by other family members or not.

I also want you to think long and hard about debt. The most common money related stress I see is being freaked out about being in the financial hole. Some spenders make a mess of their finances by maxing out their credit cards or buying into a mortgage that's over their heads or taking out a loan they're unable to pay back. Others get there due to a series of unfortunate events like unexpected medical bills, a job loss or some other catastrophe. Both Anna Koopman and Beth Arvin are good examples of the latter. Either way, you have to do your best to stay calm. Stressing about debt won't make it disappear. I find it only makes things worse. Gaining control of your situation through good planning, expert help and smarter money habits is the way to make yourself feel better.

Credit cards tend to do the most damage so I always advise my patients who struggle with debt stress to devise ways of limiting their use. Although I think all money personality types are susceptible to credit card abuse, Beginners are especially vulnerable because they don't have a lot of experience paying bills or understanding how quickly the interest on their purchases can compound. Before they know it they're in trouble. Other types need to learn impulse control and develop a sense of responsibility with their cards.

You can cut up your cards and stick with cash but I recognize that's not always practical. So to reduce credit card spending, I advise creating as many barriers to using them as possible. You might, for example, not allow websites to store your credit card information; if you have to fetch your wallet every single time you buy something online, I'll bet you'll think twice about completing the transaction. Also consider setting a spending limit before you go to the store and then write it down on your wrist so you're reminded of it every time you reach for an item. Or before you allow yourself to make a purchase, name at least five reasons why you need to buy it. Any game, rule or trick you can devise to reduce card use will keep you from sliding towards unnecessary debt and the despair that comes along with it.

Before we leave the subject of money stress, I want you to consider one more suggestion that may at first seem paradoxical. Donate to charity. Yes, I am asking you to give away some of your hard earned cash though you struggle with money stress. It's something I strongly recommend to my patients and something I'm committed to in my own life. Here's why:

Helping those less fortunate makes you think about money in a different way. I'm sure you've heard the saying that it's better to give than receive. Making a charitable contribution allows you see how money—and you—can have a positive impact on someone else's life through self-sacrifice and generosity. No matter how dire you think things are in your own life, there is always someone who is in greater need.

I understand when you have money hang ups it can be difficult to write a check that doesn't add to your personal financial wellbeing. If you're not at the point where you feel comfortable contributing from your already tight budget, consider raising money by participating in an event like a walk-a-thon or donation drive. Or spend some time doing community service. Trust me. Making someone else's life better is a wonderful, life-affirming experience that has a way of putting your money stress into perspective.

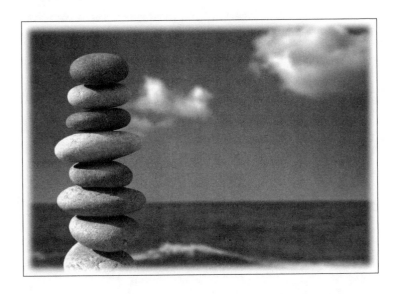

Chapter 6
Emotions and Thoughts

Savor, Shake, Sweat, and Share

Stress was everywhere in the culture and family of my childhood, and never mentioned. Our parents waged an uneasy, unspoken battle with each other—our misbehavior got us warning looks instead of correction and instruction, and disapproval was the favored method of discipline. Disappointment was met with tightened lips, anger was put away in silence, and tragedy was never mentioned again. The lesson was clear: The right way to deal with stress was to put it away inside and ignore it. Don't ask, don't tell, don't talk about it.

It's funny, and not funny, how stress grows inside you until it becomes a way of life. The more you ignore it, the harder it is to meet new stresses in any other way.

"You are so calm," my co-workers used to say to me. "Even when things are the most chaotic, you're calm and organized, and it helps us be calm too."

"What's there to worry about?" I would reply with a smile. "In a hundred years, will anyone be reading about this in the history books?" This is also what I said to myself, all the while knowing that the calmness was not quite right. My mind tiptoed around a huge pile of unmentionable things that sat in the middle of my memory, never looking, never touching. Of course I couldn't stop now, because everyone, myself included, relied on me to be calm and hold things together.

Then one day, only three days after the incredibly stressful events of September 11, 2001, I returned from the island of Maui to find that my husband, the love of my life, had moved out and left me while I was stranded in Paradise. Suddenly the pile of unmentionable things in my mind doubled and tripled, and the edges began to collapse. I went to bed and cried for four days. I barely ate. I didn't dare drink. I saw no one. I spoke to no one. I was in a precariously deep dark place, alone.

On the fifth day I showered and got dressed. I had to get out of bed because I couldn't stay there anymore. Besides, I had a date. A neighbor I didn't know well had asked me several weeks earlier to take an Italian course with her in San Francisco, and I had agreed. Today was the first class, and I was driving. I picked up Jackie, my neighbor, and we hadn't been on the road long when she asked, "How are you doing?" It was a valid question for anyone in those first days after 9/11.

As we crossed the Bay Bridge, for some reason I set aside all I had been taught my whole life, and I spilled it all—how bad I felt about the airplanes and the people who had died, how hard it had been to be so far away from home and stranded, how devastated I felt that my husband had left me as if I meant nothing to him, how angry and depressed and overwhelmed and alone I was. I cried and cried until it was hard to see to drive. When we got across the bridge I pulled off at an exit and parked the car. Jackie and I both sat there sobbing, until we stopped. Then we mopped our eyes and blew our noses, and drove on to our class. It was the first time, the very first time, I had ever shared anguish with anyone.

Once I opened up to Jackie, it became hard to close down again. Over the next weeks, and then months and years, I worked hard to heal. I saw therapists, read books, and experimented with friends. Little by little I learned new ways to face down anger and anxiety and doubt and uncertainty and disappointment, some of the underlying emotions that cause stress for me.

Here are the most important things I learned to do:

Savor.

Savor your emotion. Be glad you can feel, that you have doubt, that you care enough to feel disappointed or sad or angry. Then savor yourself, your skills, your enjoyment of life. Savor sunrises and sunsets and rain. Savor red wine and ripe peaches. Savor whatever you like.

Shake.

If you watch an animal in the wild, you will see him shake off stress after a chase or when he slips away from a predator. All animals do this—it helps them get rid of pent-up energy and the chemicals their bodies produce when they are under attack. Humans probably have the instinct to do this too, but we think it looks stupid to shake. Who cares? When you're stressed, shaking helps release tension. Go ahead, put on some dance music and shake all over.

Sweat.

Shortly after talking with my friend Jackie, I started running again and I joined a yoga class. Running had always provided a time for me to work out problems. In the past I had used this time to focus on solving work problems, but now I turned the time and skill on myself. Yoga relaxed my body and mind, so I felt strong and rested. I chanted forgiveness and love and strength and goodness. It doesn't matter how you do it, regular exercise is a terrific de-stressor. How can you be rigid and tight when you are exerting yourself to the max and sweating like a pig? While you're at it, make your mind sweat a little too. Learn something new, do something challenging that has nothing to do with the cause of your stress, stretch yourself.

Share.

Telling someone was the crucial first step I took. It helped me open up so that I could learn to manage the stress in my life in a more productive way. Now I talk more, and more honestly. A few years ago I started writing about my life. In doing so I had to think about a lot of things I had never put into words. In fact I had put some of these things away so completely that I had never actually thought about them before. When I wrote them down, I began to understand them, and the stresses around them became much weaker. A truth about stress is that it's strongest when you deny it, and it's weaker when you expose it and talk, or write, about it.

The fact is, stress is everywhere in life. It's at work and at home. It's in your family and in your community. It's on the news and in the phone call you get from your mom. Sometimes it's real, as in the loss of a job or the death of a loved one, and sometimes you make it up, as in worry about things that haven't happened yet. There's nothing shameful about stress, everyone has it. The only time stress is a shame is when you let it get the best of you, when you let stress shut you down. You don't have to do that! Savor, Shake, Sweat, and Share, and soon you'll send Stress packing. Instead of stressed, you'll feel serene. Whew, what a relief.

— Dana Hill —

Be Not Afraid

My youngest daughter and I scan the shelves of the local video store. She hands me the DVD *Just Like Heaven* that she wants to rent. I reach for the movie, but my arm doesn't feel like it's attached to my body. The floor slants under my feet. The fluorescent lights glare too brightly. My heart pounds. I glance at the other patrons. They move in slow motion. Their voices sound muffled, as though I'm hearing them through earmuffs.

I breathe deeply—in and out and in and out. I grab for my daughter's hand and give it a tight squeeze.

"A panic attack?" she whispers to me.

I nod. After nearly forty years of anxiety disorder, I know that the attack will be over soon. In a few minutes, I feel the blood rush back to my face, signaling the end of the attack. I smile at my daughter, and we walk to the checkout counter with Reese Witherspoon in hand.

I suffered my first panic attack while sitting in my eighth grade English class. I had no idea what was happening to me. The teacher was explaining subordinate clauses for the eighteenth time. Suddenly, his voice sounded far away, as if he were speaking through a cardboard tube. I touched my cheeks; they were numb. My throat tightened, and I couldn't swallow. My stomach ached.

I had to leave. I raised my hand. "I need to go to the nurse," I said. I didn't recognize the voice as my own. I raced from the classroom, convinced that I was either dying or going insane.

Day after day, I experienced these episodes in school, raced to the nurse's office, and had to be sent home. I felt safe at home, under my ballerina print quilt. I became so afraid that I refused to go to school. At first, my parents tried to reason with me. Finally, my father yelled and my mother cried, but I was too paralyzed by fear to obey.

My parents took me to a doctor who ordered a full complement of tests. I had an EKG and a neurological exam. Many vials of blood were drawn and GI X-rays were taken. The results of the tests were normal. I was physically healthy. The doctor suggested I see a psychologist. Was I losing my mind, after all?

The psychologist was a middle-aged man, who told corny jokes and made me laugh. I was at ease in his office right away and was comfortable describing my episodes to him.

"I believe you are having panic attacks. Many people experience them," he told me. "Think about an animal that is being attacked: Its body prepares to fight or run. Your body is reacting as if there's an attacker, but the threat doesn't really exist."

I was so relieved to have a name for what was happening to me and to realize that I was not alone.

My psychologist taught me deep breathing and muscle relaxation techniques to cope with the panic attacks. He had me visualize a place I felt safe in order to calm me. Sometimes, I imagined lying on the warm sands of the Jersey shore; other times, I dreamed of snuggling beneath my pastel Degas comforter.

Bit by bit, he re-introduced me to school. At first, we visited the empty classroom after hours. I sat at my desk, took full breaths, and thought about the beach and sea.

"Many people with panic disorder feel the need to escape wherever they are," my psychologist said. "Once they know they can leave, they feel more relaxed." For this reason, he convinced my teachers to allow me to exit the classroom whenever I needed.

I returned to school gradually—just mornings initially and then for full days. When the panic attacks occurred, I tried to remain in my chair and use my coping methods. Sometimes, I had to leave the room and walk the halls until the panic subsided. Each day I stayed at school was a victory, and my confidence increased. Soon, I was a regular kid again, complaining about science projects and gossiping about guys with my friends.

I have continued to use the tools my psychologist taught me decades ago. They have helped me through college and graduate school, moves across the country, and the raising of five children. However, I still have times when my anxiety causes pain.

Last spring, my second oldest daughter completed a graduate program at a college a thousand miles away. I struggled with boarding an airplane, but, in the end, I couldn't face flying at 35,000 feet without any means of escape. I missed watching proudly as she accepted her diploma; she missed having her mother cheer loudly for her from the stands.

But each day, I strive to handle my anxiety better. I know that my life is richer when I face my fears and overcome them. Recently, a fifth grade teacher asked me to speak to her class about my nonfiction books. I felt anxiety grip me as I thought about spending time in a grammar school classroom once again. I nearly said, "No," but instead I jumped in.

Toward the end of my presentation, I did have a panic attack. I fought to keep my feet rooted to the floor and concentrate on the students' questions.

"Do police dogs eat pork chops?" one child asked. I laughed, breathed deeply, and continued.

— Marie-Therese Miller —

The Panic Monster

I picked up a can of chicken noodle soup and put it in my grocery cart. I moved up the grocery aisle and felt my heart pick up speed. That's strange, I thought. I felt a little out of breath, like I'd jogged up the aisle.

It reminded me of that day months earlier at a rock concert. That hot day in the full-capacity crowd, I felt claustrophobic—heartbeat rising like the heat. My friend and I picked our way through the crowd trying to find a little room to breathe. My pulse escalated. My mind said there was nothing to fear, but my body didn't listen. Soon, my heart was racing and I needed to get out of that stadium.

Embarrassed, I told my friend and we found a stairway up and a way out. We totally missed The Rolling Stones.

I couldn't explain the anxiety I'd felt that day. It was like when I had to deliver a speech in school. Same escalating heartbeat. Same shortness of breath. Same shakiness. But there was no speech and no class. I loved rock and roll and concerts where I could disappear in the crowd, relax, and enjoy. Now this strange panic was invading my life even at a rock concert, even in a grocery store. I didn't know why. I just wanted to keep it under control until I could pick up some fruit and get through the checkout lane.

The store was nearly empty. The one cashier moved dreadfully slow. My heart beat dreadfully fast. I felt dizzy. My chest ached. I was sweating. Was I having a heart attack? I was only twenty years old. What was happening to me? I wasn't going to make it through the checkout line. I wheeled my grocery cart to the back of the store, abandoned it, and ducked out the exit.

In my car the symptoms began to dissipate. I felt wrung out like I'd just run a marathon. "What is wrong with me?" I cried out loud, pounding the steering wheel.

In the following months I felt panic rise in restaurants and movie theaters. When I was out with friends, I struggled to keep the panic under control. I learned a couple of drinks helped contain the panic monster that lurked beneath the surface waiting to attack. Claustrophobia was the best explanation I could come up with, but I didn't need to be closed in to feel it.

I was embarrassed to tell anyone. How could I explain my intense anxiety in a grocery store? I searched for help. When my fiancé and I were planning our wedding, the church advertised their new counseling ministry. I made an appointment. The lady, God bless her, didn't know how to help me except to pray. Okay, but I needed more.

When I went for my blood test to get our marriage license, I tried to explain my experiences to the doctor. "Is there something you can give me to help me stay calm enough to get through the wedding?" I asked. He gave me a prescription. On my wedding day, it was no help. I'm now convinced it was a placebo.

A few years later another doctor told me I had mitral valve prolapse syndrome—a problem with a valve in the heart that can cause the heart to start racing. I'd heard about it on the news, but no other doctor has ever detected a problem with my heart.

My husband's job took us to a new town and I heard about counseling at the local mental health center. I went. The counselor talked with me at length about what I felt, about my childhood traumas. But the panic persisted. I constantly felt stressed.

Then one day I turned on the television and heard a man saying, "... escalating heartbeat, chest pain, shortness of breath, shaking, sweating. It feels like you're having a heart attack, and many people think that's what's happening. It feels like you're dying, but these episodes are not harmful."

You mean I wasn't the only one? Astounded, I wanted to hug the TV! That TV talk show guest used the term "panic attack" and I knew immediately that's what I'd been experiencing. It had a name!

Then I met Betty. She talked about her struggles with "anxiety disorder." Suddenly someone I knew experienced this! We quickly became friends. Betty took prescription meds to manage her panic disorder, though she hated that she needed them.

I learned from a National Institute of Mental Health brochure (1994) that there are different kinds of anxiety disorders, including generalized anxiety disorder, panic disorder, social phobia, agoraphobia, obsessive-compulsive disorder, and post-traumatic stress disorder. Many people fear public speaking, but it's a "disorder" when it affects your life, your career—when you pass up a promotion because you can't give a presentation, when you purposely lose so you don't have to give the winner's speech. I guessed mine was either social or panic disorder.

I learned it's possible to de-sensitize to panic triggers. Agoraphobics, who can become prisoners in their homes, for example, can take baby steps: step outside for a moment. Next time, take two steps.

Experts said fighting the symptoms only makes them escalate. Don't fight them. Let it happen. Like that's easy! But I tried, and practiced, and began to see progress.

But I also experienced setbacks. A Bible study required participants to introduce themselves. As my turn grew closer, my heart rate escalated. I struggled to breathe. Too shaky to move, too breathless to speak, I finally excused myself and headed for the door, my knees so weak I feared I wouldn't make it out. That setback haunted me for years and to this day reminds me the panic monster is lurking, waiting to pounce.

Today, I haven't had a panic attack in years. My writing career has gained momentum and I've been asked to speak. In my past I never dreamed I'd say yes, but I have. The more I do it, the easier it becomes.

Three years ago I joined Toastmasters, a peer group that gives training and practice in public speaking, which has further helped me conquer the panic monster.

A few weeks ago I attended a conference for professional writers and speakers as a new member. After I signed up I learned everyone had to introduce themselves! Had I known before I made my travel arrangements, I might have passed on the conference. During dinner, one by one each table was called up on stage before the room of nearly one hundred professional speakers and writers. I stood in line. I gripped my new book. I walked to the microphone. And I did it! Then I returned to my seat.

As I sat there, I marveled, remembering the times my heart pounded just sitting in a restaurant and when I couldn't remain calm enough to say my name to a group of twelve women in a Bible study. Yet I was in a group of professional speakers having dinner, feeling relaxed, and actually enjoying the conversation. Baby steps have carried me a long way. And daily I'm conquering the panic monster.

~ Dianne E. Butts ~

Emotions and Thoughts

Introduction

In the preceding chapters we discussed some of the major causes of stress. Now I'd like to talk about what effect stress can have on you, then talk about how you might change your thinking in order to lead a less stressful life.

As you can see in the stories included in this chapter, there's a lengthy laundry list of physical and psychological responses to living a stressful existence. Some happen in the short term. Others are more insidious. The truth is your body and mind can react similarly no matter what type of stress you're under. That's right: A bride planning a wedding and a man going through a divorce can be susceptible to the same range of symptoms.

For some, stress rises up from a sudden incident. As a result, your body might perceive that quick change as a threat where the immediate reaction is one of flight or fight. The choice is to stand there and boldly take on your aggressor or run like the wind. Any time something seems life threatening even for an instant, your stomach drops and your heart jumps. For example, you'll have an involuntary response anytime there's a sudden slam of car brakes, your chair slips unexpectedly or you accidentally cut your finger with a knife. You may also have a similar reaction in circumstances that are uncomfortable though clearly not dangerous. If you get stage fright before giving a speech or dread socializing at parties you know exactly what I mean.

As for what causes that familiar edgy feeling, you have your sympathetic nervous system to thank for that. When you're hit with a stress, the nervous system signals the adrenal glands to release a flood of the stress hormones adrenaline and cortisol into the blood stream to elevate heart rate, breathing rate, blood pressure, and metabolism. Your blood vessels open wider to allow more blood flow to large muscle groups in case they're needed to flee the scene. For the same reason, your liver releases some of its stored glucose for a shot of instant energy. Your pupils dilate to sharpen your vision and your sweat glands produce sweat to cool your body. (A panic attack is at the extreme end of this reaction arc.)

All of these physical reactions prepare you to better handle a threat quickly and effectively. Clearly flight or fight response was useful to our ancestors when they were at risk of being eaten by a mountain lion. However, it's useful for us modern folks too. A little burst of nervous energy every now and then might just enhance your ability to perform well under pressure; it keeps you on your toes, ready to respond to all sorts of everyday challenges, from problems at the office to issues at home. And when the nervous system quickly returns to its normal state at a lower level of function and powers down in appropriate moments, there's no harm done.

Problems arise if stress is ongoing. High stress conditions that are long lasting produce a sustained fight-or-flight response that asks the nervous system to stay continually activated at low levels in order to keep up with a ceaseless stream of stress-induced emotions. Ultimately, this leaves you feeling depleted and overwhelmed.

Long-term stress is associated with just about every physical and psychological ailment you can name. The American Institute of Stress publishes a list of the most common symptoms, including headaches, teeth grinding, weight gain, weight loss, insomnia, frequent urination, difficulty concentrating, mood swings, lack of sexual desire—and these are just a few among the first fifty on the list! By the way, I talk more about the effects of stress and how to manage them in my book *Chicken Soup for the Soul: Think Positive for Great Health* (September 2012).

Stress left unaddressed can lead to serious, debilitating health issues. Depression, anxiety, heart attacks, stroke, hypertension, gastrointestinal disorders, skin conditions and rheumatoid arthritis all have links to continuing stress. High stress levels have also been associated with immune system disturbances that increase susceptibility to infections, a host of viral disorders ranging from the common cold and herpes to AIDS and certain cancers, as well as autoimmune diseases such as rheumatoid arthritis and multiple sclerosis and degenerative neurological disorders such as Parkinson's disease.

Psychological disorders such as clinical depression, anxiety and addiction are also thought to have a stress related component. In many cases, however, this is a chicken or egg relationship when it comes to knowing which exacerbates which. In fact, I'd be hard pressed to think of any ailment that stress doesn't aggravate. As scientists learn more about the toll stress takes on the body and mind, the list will undoubtedly keep on growing.

Thought Traps

The experience of stress is difficult for scientists to define because it is a highly subjective phenomenon. We all have our own unique stress profiles. For example, Dana Hill certainly seems to handle stress much differently than the other two storytellers in this chapter. Something distressful for one individual may be no sweat for another. Everyone responds to pressure differently too. Some people take it in stride, while others fall apart over every paper cut and minor insult. Some people blush, some eat more, while others grow pale or eat less. Some turn to alcohol or drugs to deal with their discomfort while others go for a run or hit the gym. Virtually any reaction to stress you can think of is a possibility. Our concern is developing the healthiest responses to your emotions.

I believe people who have a chronic problem with managing stress may have an inaccurate perception of reality. What I mean by this is that they hold a distorted view of themselves, circumstances and the world. No matter what their situation, they let their thoughts lead their emotions to a dark place.

One classic irrational thought pattern is sometimes referred to as "catastrophizing" or "awfulizing." This is when you allow your mind to imagine only the worst possible outcome for a situation; imaginary consequences are usually far more terrible than what could ever happen. For instance, a parent may believe that every small mistake he makes in raising his children is proof that he's a terrible parent. Or a lawyer starts to believe that she is completely incompetent and her practice will never grow, simply because she lost one case. This sort of thinking takes a current situation and gives it the most negative spin possible.

Fortune telling, another common thinking error, is basically the same sort of worst case thinking except that it projects worry into the future without centering on the present. Fortune tellers anticipate everything that can go wrong will go wrong, thus they start feeling anxiety even before an event happens — if it ever does. While it isn't humanly possible to predict the future, when you believe something is about to go wrong it can affect your performance. Think of an employee who believes he won't get a raise. In his mind, his request has been shot down before he's ever made it. Plus the anxiety and worry that go along with mentally rehearsing his failure over and over again is exhausting and stressful.

Rethinking Your Thoughts

You may have the impression that thoughts are spun from thin air and magically pop into your head just like thought bubbles in the Sunday comics. You may also believe you have no control over how they form or travel through your mind. In actuality, thoughts are something you create. That's good news if you're prone to inaccurate thinking. When you get used to thinking certain thoughts in a certain way, negativity can easily become a bad habit, much like biting your nails, smoking or using a fork as a back scratcher. It's possible, however, to guide your thoughts down a sunnier path.

Since you are the architect of your own thoughts, you get

to lay the blueprints for the thoughts you'd like to have. If you believe you may have a self-defeating inner dialog going on in your head, you can try stopping negative thoughts in their tracks by becoming aware of them. One way to analyze the tenor of your personal narrative is by keeping a thought journal. Pay attention to the specific thoughts you have, the circumstances under which you have them, and associated emotions. Record your thoughts as frequently as you can, as close to the time you have them and in as much detail as possible. Do this for up to a week (but even a day or two can be instructive). When you step back and look at the flow of your thoughts as a whole you will undoubtedly see distinct patterns emerge. Then you'll have an inkling about the people, places and things that most commonly stimulate your erroneous thinking—and most importantly, how you can go about changing them.

Once you've isolated the thought patterns that hold you back and dial up your stress, you can begin addressing them. I tell my patients to look for objective, measurable evidence that a thought is realistic. For example, if you have never been in an elevator that has crashed to the basement—despite your best catastrophizing to the contrary—that's a pretty good indication it isn't likely to happen the next time or the time after that. Pretty soon it dawns on you that the more reasonable expectation is an uneventful trip to the floor of your choice.

Understanding your thought habits provides you with an opportunity to edit them. Every time you catch yourself catastrophizing, fortune telling or engaging in some other unproductive thinking, picture a broom sweeping the thought away and a breeze blowing in a more rational thought. (The broom and breeze are only suggestions; you may use any imagery you wish.) In this way you can sweep out a thought like, "The elevator is going to crash and I'm going to die!" and allow the breeze to blow in a more helpful thought such as, "No, that's not true. This elevator has never had a serious maintenance issue. The ride up to the seventh floor will be smooth and quick, just like always."

I don't want to represent to you that swapping irrational thoughts for rational ones is an instantaneous process. Panic attacks like those described in this chapter can take a long while to get under control, even when you seek medical attention. It takes a conscious, concentrated effort, not to mention a lot of time, practice, and patience. Still, if you commit to better thought management, you can replace a good portion of your stressful thoughts with more productive ones. In working with clients, and in my own life, I've come to the conclusion that making the effort to alter the general trend of irrational thoughts is a more realistic goal than trying to banish inaccurate thinking completely all at once. It's not possible for anyone to sail through life without ever having another irrational thought.

Keep in mind too, that even emotions you may have labeled undesirable have their purpose. Anger, sadness, disgust and other feelings with generally negative connotations are a valid part of the normal human experience. It's appropriate to feel disgust when you taste spoiled milk and it's okay to feel sad when you lose someone you love. When you witness your child fall down or have an encounter with an angry boss, feeling a bit of stress and anxiety makes sense. An emotion only causes trouble when you blow it out of proportion or begin experiencing it so frequently it becomes the norm. Having control over your emotions helps control stress.

Radical Acceptance

Before we leave the topic of stress and emotions, I want to introduce you to one other concept therapists have come to see as having value for managing stress and unconstructive thinking. A popular therapeutic approach to managing emotion is called Dialectical Behavior Therapy (DBT). Within a set of tools offered by DBT is the idea of radical acceptance, which means that you accept life and reality as it's given to you and you don't continue to struggle with solving the problem in an unhealthy way. This doesn't mean standing by as bad things happen in your life. It means accepting that "it is what it is" and making a choice to do the best you can.

Perhaps your challenges in life have been enormous and this has affected you deeply. Maybe your parents divorced when you were young and you feel your childhood was stolen from you, you had a terrible accident, or you've been the victim of theft. All of these things are unfortunate and can conjure up strong emotions. With radical acceptance, you accept the circumstances that have led you to where you are on a deep level. You make no judgment about whether things are right or wrong. They just are. You may never fully understand why something happened to you the way it did but it no longer matters. Instead of staying in an emotional hole as a result of a trauma, you make the choice to heal and move on.

In my work, I've seen radical acceptance work wonders. People who learn to be gentle with themselves are able to stop being so self-critical and even learn to love themselves. Once they do that, they are able to practice the same spirit of acceptance and forgiveness with other people too. They soon realize that it's not the size or severity of a problem that allows them to accept it as is. It's their willingness to learn about how to deal with stress differently.

Turn the page to see the American Institute of Stress's Top 50 Most Common Signs and Symptoms of Stress.

American Institute of Stress's Top 50 Most Common Signs and Symptoms of Stress

1.	Frequent headaches, jaw clenching or pain
2.	Gritting, grinding teeth
3.	Stuttering or stammering
4.	Tremors, trembling of lips, hands
5.	Neck ache, back pain, muscle spasms
6.	Light headedness, faintness, dizziness
7.	Ringing, buzzing or "popping" sounds
8.	Frequent blushing, sweating
9.	Cold or sweaty hands, feet
10.	Dry mouth, problems swallowing
11.	Frequent colds, infections, herpes sores
12.	Rashes, itching, hives, "goose bumps"
13.	Unexplained or frequent "allergy" attacks
14.	Heartburn, stomach pain, nausea
15.	Excess belching, flatulence
16.	Constipation, diarrhea
17.	Difficulty breathing, sighing
18.	Sudden attacks of panic
19.	Chest pain, palpitations
20.	Frequent urination
21.	Poor sexual desire or performance
22.	Excess anxiety, worry, guilt, nervousness
23.	Increased anger, frustration, hostility
24.	Depression, frequent or wild mood swings

25. Increased or decreased appetite
26. Insomnia, nightmares, disturbing dreams
27. Difficulty concentrating, racing thoughts
28. Trouble learning new information
29. Forgetfulness, disorganization, confusion
30. Difficulty in making decisions
31. Feeling overloaded or overwhelmed
32. Frequent crying spells or suicidal thoughts
33. Feelings of loneliness or worthlessness
34. Little interest in appearance, punctuality
35. Nervous habits, fidgeting, feet tapping
36. Increased frustration, irritability, edginess
37. Overreaction to petty annoyances
38. Increased number of minor accidents
39. Obsessive or compulsive behavior
40. Reduced work efficiency or productivity
41. Lies or excuses to cover up poor work
42. Rapid or mumbled speech
43. Excessive defensiveness or suspiciousness
44. Problems in communication, sharing
45. Social withdrawal and isolation
46. Constant tiredness, weakness, fatigue
47. Frequent use of over-the-counter drugs
48. Weight gain or loss without diet
49. Increased smoking, alcohol or drug use
50. Excessive gambling or impulse buying

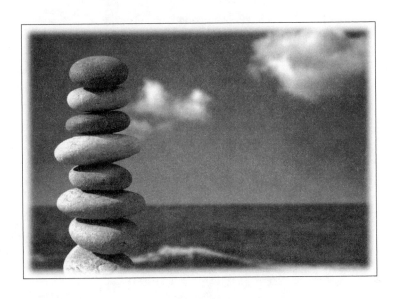

Chapter 7
Mind Your Stress

The Gratitude Antidote

Christmas. The most glorious time of the year. But Christmas this past year was anything but glorious for me. I had just learned that my sister's ovarian cancer had returned—for the third time. As if that weren't enough, my married son, Rob, called and told my husband Larry and me that his wife had deserted him and their two young sons. There was, he said between sobs, no chance that she would change her mind.

One week before Christmas Larry and I were on a red-eye flight to Detroit to help Rob.

I knew I was in danger of sinking into depression. I suffer from chemical depression, which can be triggered by stress. Not surprisingly, my stress level was at an all-time high.

On the plane, I said a silent prayer, asking the Lord for His guidance. "I don't know if I can make it through this," I said. Though the words were uttered only in my heart, I knew the Lord heard my plea.

The words appeared in my mind, as clear as though God had spoken to me aloud. "Be grateful."

Be grateful? What did I have to be grateful about?

The voice came again, more sternly this time. "Be grateful."

"How?" I asked.

"Be grateful and then share that gratitude with others."

In that hazy state between wakefulness and sleep, I wondered if I had imagined the entire conversation. We arrived in Detroit, exhausted and sick at heart, but determined to support Rob, who was in a state of shock.

While I took care of our grandchildren, ages six and three, Larry helped Rob find a lawyer. It was a heartbreaking process. Still, we tried to put a good face on things for the children's sake.

The boys were too young to comprehend everything, but they knew something was wrong. "Mommy doesn't live here any more," the older one told me. It took everything I had not to give way to tears.

In between caring for my grandsons and doing some much-needed housecleaning, I started writing a list of blessings. "Okay," I told the Lord. "I'm doing my best to be grateful. How do I share it with others?"

"Start a blog."

"A blog?" I have no technical skills and am fortunate to be able to send e-mail.

"Write about your gratitude. You can touch the lives of others."

By now I had learned not to argue with the Voice.

I mulled over the Lord's instructions. Could I do it? In the midst of one of the darkest times of my life, I decided that I would write every day for a year about a blessing.

After Rob found a lawyer and we had things on a better footing for him, we returned to our home in Colorado where we spent Christmas Day with our other children. The following day, Larry and I drove to Utah where I spent the next three weeks with my sister, staying with her while she went through the first session of chemotherapy.

I started my blog on New Year's Day, while in Utah. Early each morning, before the rest of the household stirred, I posted a short message, writing about something for which I was grateful. My subjects focused on simple, everyday blessings. A sunny day during the long dark month of January. An eighteen-year-old car that still runs.

Nearly six months have passed since I started "The Gratitude Project." The depression I dreaded failed to materialize. The stress remained, but I was able to deal with it, doing what was necessary for my sister in addition to taking care of the housework and helping to care for her three-year-old granddaughter who lives with her.

Stress is a part of our lives. Few, if any of us, can get through this life without experiencing some degree of stress and its attendant consequences. But I learned that it is manageable. With the Lord's help, I found a way to find joy in the midst of darkness.

~ Jane McBride Choate ~

Ripple Effect

When I was seven, my family moved into a newer, bigger house to fit our growing family. The best feature, though, was not the house's size, nor the fact that I would get my own bedroom instead of having to share with my sister. It was the small creek just down the hill in the woods behind the house. Even then, I recognized its significance.

While my siblings and I spent our childhood playing in the woods beside the creek, I never took time to stay still and observe the water. Being a teenager changed that. The creek became my refuge.

I would come home after a stressful school day and walk straight down the hill. I would balance from stone to stone until I reached a big boulder in the middle of the creek, and there I would sit and write in my journal, the water bubbling around me.

Countless times, I ran down that hill to escape a fight with my parents. I'd sit on one of the stones and cry as I watched the water. But something about the sound of the water, its continual sloshy flow, slowed my tears. I found myself watching the tiny ripples, thinking about how there were so many of them that you couldn't begin to count, how they constantly, consistently appeared. Even with all its activity, the creek had a steadiness, and it steadied me.

Now I am an adult in New York City, and my location makes it hard to hold onto any kind of calm. Busy people constantly surround me, blocking the sidewalks and crowding the subway cars, and the fever pitch of their hurry is contagious.

On one very stressful day, I called my trusted friend Sara during lunch. I was sitting on a bench in Madison Square Park and tons of people were walking by, but I couldn't stop my tears. My ex was in town, I told my friend, and I explained how the ex managed to make me happy one minute and angry in the next. My co-worker got a promotion, I said, and I was happy for her in theory, but seeing her in a new position freaked me out about my own job. Was I performing well enough?

"You can't hold onto these feelings," said Sara. "I mean, don't be mad at yourself—we can't help feeling the way we feel sometimes. But you can't carry your jealousy and anger around and let it stress you out. You have to let it go."

"I know that," I said. "But I don't know how. How do you just drop feelings? How do you let them go?"

"I don't know," said Sara. "Maybe you need to meditate or something."

Meditating seemed as good an idea as any. I hung up the phone, prepared to take a few deep breaths before heading back to the office. I tried to think of an image to hold in my head while I breathed. Something that signified calm.

Then I let out my breath and laughed. I was sitting right in front of a fountain! I approached it, remembering the creek that had helped me growing up. The water spouted from the top of the fountain and fell into the pool below, creating a million ripples that flowed into each other as new ones appeared. Water was steady—it didn't disappear, but it was constantly changing. I needed to go with the flow, to let myself change.

I walked back to work calmer than before, grinning at almost-forgotten memories.

— Eve Legato —

My Eight Gets

He was sixty-seven years old. His factory—and everything he had worked for his entire life—had gone up in flames. Yet, Thomas Edison looked at the ruins and said, "There's value in disaster. All our mistakes are burned up. Thank God, we can start anew."

That's what I call a positive attitude. And I've found a positive attitude vital for handling stress with calm confidence.

For most of my life, I have battled depression. Though it's not as obvious as a broken leg, it's just as painful, and it disrupts life, decreases productivity, and contributes to marital and job stress.

"This is more than I can handle." That's what I told myself for years; but it wasn't true for me, just as it wasn't true for great leaders and strong men like Abraham Lincoln who fought the same battle.

While you can't talk yourself out of depression any more than you can talk yourself out of diabetes or cancer, I've learned how positive self talk can improve coping skills. A positive attitude is an important element of half a dozen stress-busting strategies I practice, which I call my "Eight Gets."

When I begin to feel stressed and overwhelmed, the first thing I do is GET FOCUSED. Instead of thinking about bills, a broken down car, or bad hair days, I make a conscious effort to flood my brain with positive, hopeful thoughts such as "I can get through this. I have what it takes to deal with whatever I need to handle. I'm confident of my abilities."

Simply telling yourself good things is empowering. I wrote a list of affirmations such as "I am relaxed and worry free. I enjoy life and choose to be happy." Even if the statements aren't currently true or I don't really believe them, my mind eventually comes to believe what I tell it, so I tell it I am already the type of person I want to become. Focusing on the positive, rather than on worries, keeps stress at bay.

My second step in relieving stress is GET FRIENDLY. Connecting with others is a great tranquilizer. A phone call, lunch with a friend, or kisses from your significant other are fun and free prescriptions for a brighter outlook. This helps me slide right into my third "get," which is GET GIGGLING.

Watching funny movies or playing with children is a fantastic mood lifter. I enjoy my grandson because with him I can let go of inhibitions. We dance and sing, wear funny glasses with mustaches, and make up silly rhymes. When I'm stressed and need to smile, I pull out some photos of us. Laughing and smiling release endorphins in your brain. These are chemicals that make you feel good. Chocolate does the same thing, but a good laugh is less fattening.

A friend of mine, who had a very frustrating job, told me that one day she was inspired by a co-worker, so she decided to emulate that woman and smile at everyone she encountered. Right away, she found herself less frustrated and more at peace. "It sounds corny," she told me, "but smiling works!"

My fourth suggestion is GET RHYTHM.

Positive, upbeat tunes help relieve stress too. Singing and dancing or just tapping my toes sends a message to my brain that I'm relaxed and happy. Rather than complaining about what stresses me, I break out my old CDs and try to remember the words to songs I loved in high school.

Another important stress busting measure is to GET BUSY.

There is a famous quote that goes something like "The best way to lift yourself up is to bend down and help someone else." We all need to feel like we're involved in something significant outside ourselves. I've enjoyed volunteering at a food pantry and a women's shelter. As a result, I discovered that contentment and joy boomerang. Give them away and they bounce back to you. Making life better for others will elevate your self-esteem as well as your mood.

Number six on my list is GET PHYSICAL.

There are two elements to this one. Both physical exercise and physical contact, like a massage or a hug are good for mental health. A walk with a friend is the perfect combination. The beauty of nature, fresh air, good conversation and exercise can soothe the toughest stress. And taking my dog along is even more relaxing. Watching his ears flop as he bounces down the road always brings a smile to my face.

Exercise and physical closeness both affect brain chemicals; so don't just jog, hug somebody—anybody, everybody! A hug reduces tension, lowers blood pressure, and boosts your immunity to illness. They feel good, they make people happy, and they're free! They're healthy for the "hugger" as well as the "hugee."

Shhhh. A very important technique for relieving stress is to GET QUIET.

Our lives are so busy, we rarely take the time to get away and relax, even if it's just for half an hour or fifteen minutes. Balance is essential to stress free living. Being busy and connecting with others can be great, but sometimes I need to kick back with a good book on my porch swing, listen to the birds sing, and enjoy the solitude.

Last, but not least, we need to GET THANKFUL.

In our busy world, it takes a conscious effort to count our blessings. A frazzled attitude of discontent and frustration has a hard time competing with an attitude of gratitude.

For years, I've practiced these eight simple tools to deal with depression, but they're useful for anyone with any type of stress. If you're discouraged or you need to refresh your soul, I suggest trying what I do. Close your eyes, take a few deep breaths, and refocus on the more positive things in life.

— Marsha Mott Jordan —

Mind Your Stress

Introduction

Since you're reading a book about how to reduce stress, I assume you've decided it's time to get serious about managing your own stress level. To help you in this worthwhile pursuit, all of the other chapters in this book include numerous proactive steps you can take to help relieve tension and anxiety. However, in this chapter, I advocate doing nothing.

Yes, that's right. Do Nothing. Sit there, close your eyes and let your mind go blank. Be like Eve Legato and mesmerize yourself with flowing water. Get off the daily merry-go-round for just a few minutes. Proof is mounting that clearing away mental clutter and letting go of your emotions can have a profoundly positive effect on your wellbeing. We are just beginning to understand how the mind and body influence each other and how shaping that relationship with activities like meditation, spirituality and positive thinking can help manage stress. The more science discovers, the more we realize what a valuable complement to your other stress reduction efforts these practices can be.

Ohm Ohm Good

When you think of meditation, it may conjure up images of monks sitting cross-legged on a mountaintop, chanting their way to spiritual enlightenment. The average person doesn't need to practice this style of meditation. The literal meaning of the word meditation is awareness. So whatever you do to achieve awareness can be considered meditation. It can indeed be sitting cross-legged on a mountaintop but it can also take the form of a contemplative yoga class, a relaxation DVD or simply finding a moment to concentrate on your breath.

Meditation can be anything you do for the purpose of slowing down the constant chatter in your head. One common technique involves concentrating on a single point of focus to direct your thoughts away from negative thinking. If the mind wanders, you gently lead it back to its focus. You might, for instance, repeat a single word that has some special meaning to you or chant a soothing sound such as "ohm." Some people prefer to have an object, color or the rhythm of their own breath as a focal point.

In certain meditation practices, the goal is to sweep bad thoughts from the mind to create an empty space that can be filled with peace and serenity or with positive and productive thoughts. In other meditation practices, the emphasis is on mindfulness. This is the commitment to stay in the moment without passing judgment. With a mindful practice, you don't attempt to send negative thoughts away; instead, you quietly watch them flow through your mind like a bubbling stream. The mindful experience is sometimes described as "being, not doing," because it is about observation, not reaction. Similar to the concept of radical acceptance which I discussed in Chapter 6, the purpose is to witness the here and now and accept it for what it is.

Whatever the emphasis, studies find meditation can have

remarkable benefits. It appears to boost the immune system, enhance sleep quality, increase self-awareness and self-control, reduce anxiety and depressive symptoms—I could fill an entire book listing all its health advantages. And you benefit from the first moment you close your eyes and breathe deeply. An immediate response is a reduction of the stress hormones cortisol and adrenaline, as well as the release of happiness hormones like serotonin which causes your heart rate to slow, blood pressure to drop and tension to melt away. Imaging studies show structural changes to the areas of the brain associated with fear, emotion, self-control and focus after as little as 11 hours of meditation training. When you meditate consistently over a long period of time, the research also suggests you can make significant improvements in how you perceive and manage stress that is reflected in both structural brain changes and in your behavior.

Since most of us can't get away for a three-month retreat, the really good news is that even a few minutes of meditation a day can make a difference. I've had people tell me they've tried meditation but gave it up because they couldn't stop their thoughts from racing even for a few breaths. If you feel that way, keep trying. Meditation has been shown to help with stress whether you are "good at it" or not. If you revisit the practice consistently, you will get better at it over time.

If you aren't a meditator, you may want to try for short periods of time—five or ten minutes to start. Of course like anything else, the more you do it, the more you get out of it. Regular meditators tell me that every little bit helps. You can learn some techniques by attending a formal meditation or yoga class but if you'd prefer to "Ohm alone" there are dozens of other resources for learning the basics. For instance, numerous websites offer step-by-step guides and there are many high quality (and free!) how-to podcasts and YouTube videos.

Adding Spirituality

Deep religious beliefs have been long associated with lower rates of heart disease, stroke, metabolic disorders, autoimmune disease and mental health issues. For example, a University of Toronto study recently found that believing in a higher power can help block anxiety when under stress. This connection between spirituality and health comes as no surprise to those who have strong faith.

Why does belief in an almighty deity lead to health benefits? It's not entirely known. Skeptics point to flaws in the studies and surveys — for instance, the fact that religious people may simply lead less risky lifestyles than non-believers, or that very sick people are unable to attend religious services. Other critics chalk up the benefit to a placebo effect: If you trust that faith and prayer can heal you, then they will help you heal despite conferring no medical benefit. All of these criticisms are countered by a slew of recent work that accounts for these factors yet still finds religion has a protective effect in currently healthy people. And that's good news.

Whatever it can or can't do for other aspects of your health, it seems abundantly true that religious faith creates a more stress resistant physiological profile. Two factors that help people see their lives as less stressful are: 1) faith, which seems to promote an increased sense of purpose, and 2) belief in giving control to a higher power who in turn watches over you. Plus, the positive emotions associated with such belief shift thinking to be more positive overall. When your inner voice is more optimistic you're better prepared to look on the bright side and steer clear of emotional distress.

Attitude Is Everything

So, whether you arrive there by religion, therapy or by keeping a gratitude journal like Jane McBride Choate, positive thinking is one of the most powerful weapons you have in the fight against stress. As a psychologist, this is a topic that is very near and dear to my heart. I've seen how very harmful negative, anxious and depressive thinking can be. It keeps the flight-or-fight mechanisms of the body turned on far too often and for far too long and this has a way of wearing down your mental and physical defenses.

Optimism defeats stress. In the first place, believing everything will turn out fine at least opens you up to the possibility everything will work out for the better, something negative thinking doesn't even allow you to consider. According to research, optimism seems to help the body repair the stress related damage at the cellular level, seems to reduce inflammation and seems to lower levels of stress hormones. It might also dampen nervous system activity. So, instead of enduring a constant flight-or-fight feeling, you get a chance to experience the opposite "rest-and-digest" state of mind.

Not everyone is a born optimist of course. But as I've mentioned throughout these pages, there are numerous ways you can shift the tone of your thinking. (Meditation, for example!) Even the darkest thinkers are capable of calling up positive thoughts once in a while and if it helps motivate you, studies show the worst pessimists have the most to gain by trying to change their outlook on life. The more negative you are to begin with, the better positive thinking will work on reducing your stress levels.

A good place to start is with yourself. High "self enhancers"—those who perceive themselves more kindly than others do—have more advantageous cardiovascular responses to stress, bounce back faster from bad luck, and have lower baseline levels of cortisol than people who don't give themselves a break. Something as simple as jotting down a few self-affirmative statements can make an immediate difference. Changing your thinking is not only an excellent way to manage stress, research has confirmed again and again the power of healthy thinking. For now, you can focus on your thinking and see if you can reduce stress by adopting a more positive worldview.

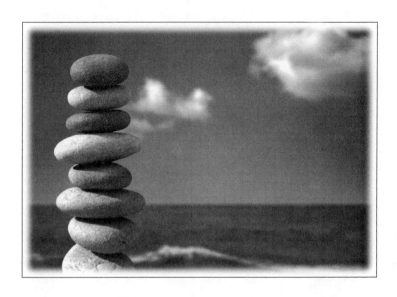

Chapter 8
De-stress
Your Lifestyle

Hear Me,
Says My Body

The effects of my husband's job loss had kicked into overdrive. We had four growing sons with growing needs. Our budget was stretched to the limit and the only working soul in our household was me. We had to cut way back on our spending just to make ends meet. I became resentful and angry at the fact that I had to work and that my husband was at home with our sons. In my heart, that was the place I always wanted to be: at home with our kids.

My husband didn't take the transition well either, at least during the first few years. He went through a period of depression and withdrawal. I tried my best to help pull him through that difficult time. Finally, he regained enough confidence to return to college to pursue an MBA degree online. Having an undergraduate degree in chemical engineering with a master's in business was a combination major corporations couldn't resist, right? Wrong. He filled out what seemed like hundreds of job applications, all to no avail.

It was a major switch for my husband, going from the left-brain-thinking engineer type to "Mr. Mom." Being at home didn't naturally agree with him and our home showed it. I would return from work with a smile on my face until I walked in. My home was barely recognizable because certain rooms were in such disarray. I would find myself screaming, asking why the house was such a mess and what my husband had been doing all day.

As time passed and my husband's job hunting continued, my stress level maxed out. One morning I woke up and could barely move my neck. Sharp pains shot up and down my neck and back. I went from general practitioner, to chiropractor, to medical therapist, and to massage therapist over the course of about five years to find relief. Major muscle spasms and trigger points had built up in my neck and shoulder muscles. My trap (trapezius) muscles were literally trapped.

Even in the midst of pain I had to continue my 120-mile roundtrip commute to work. Nothing else was coming in to support our family. I even tried to start my own businesses on the side.

My body continued to send out messages that it was overstressed, and I ignored them. But my wake-up call came when I learned my blood pressure had gone from low to borderline high. I finally began to listen to my body, and that's where my self-discovery journey began. I was determined to find the true source of my stress.

I researched sources and triggers of high blood pressure. My goal was to control my blood pressure naturally. I learned that nutrition could play a major role in elevating blood pressure, especially if your body is sensitive to sodium. I wasn't overweight and I exercised regularly, so I cut back on my sodium intake and increased the potassium and magnesium in my daily diet. Still, there were no major improvements in my blood pressure.

My health didn't truly change until I became more self-aware. I began to notice how my body responded when I reacted to things that upset me or when I was under pressure to meet a deadline or expectation. My neck, shoulder, and back muscles would tense and tighten up. I learned that I needed to refocus my thoughts and attention on things I had the power to control. You can't control people, only influence them with your own actions. I stopped focusing as much on what my husband did or did not do, and I tried my best not to focus on our income. I began to focus on what I could change, such as my mindset, my thoughts, my attitude, and my actions.

My eyes were opened once again while reading a book about stress and adrenaline. My extremely busy schedule and task-driven personality kept my adrenaline constantly going. I had been operating on high doses of adrenaline for such an extended period of time that it distressed my body. Knowing when to allow an adrenaline rush and when to switch it off is essential for stress management. And I learned I can choose whether I want the adrenaline rush to continue.

I learned that my muscle tension and blood pressure issues were all related and stemmed from the same source. The effects of too much adrenaline, in both good and bad stressful situations, had taken their toll on my body. Blood pressure screams at you if the cumulative effects of stress get out of control; your muscles lock up and cause pain to get your attention.

Over time I developed my personal health regimen. It

involves weekly weight circuit training, daily breathing and re-laxation techniques, daily visualization and mindset manage-ment. In doing this, I have reached my health goals. I lowered my blood pressure naturally. My muscle tightness, soreness, and pain are greatly reduced and controllable. At the time of writing this, my husband is still "Mr. Mom." We both learned to adjust and make the best of our circumstances. During my journey, I also discovered a love for writing, teaching, and for sharing with others what helped me overcome adversity and achieve my goals.

I can say with confidence that how I managed stress was the main source of all my physical health problems. I'm glad I was able to say goodbye to stress, because now I know how to respond whenever it decides to pay me a visit.

— Rachel L. Moore —

Power Walk

I could manage for a year and a half—I knew I could. I was tough; I had survived worse situations.

We live on Vancouver Island, and my husband had to work in Vancouver, British Columbia, three hours away, for a year and half. Three hours doesn't sound like a lot, but an hour-and-forty-five-minute ferry ride distanced us. He would stay in Vancouver during the week, and come home on weekends. We could do it; I could do it. Heck, there were single mothers and fathers out there who had spent much longer managing solely on their own, without a weekend's reprieve. This was nothing.

That year and a half tested my family and me. I was overwhelmed with the feeling that everything and everyone relied solely on me. It wreaked havoc on my stress levels and my sleep. I had started a new full-time job a few months before, so exhaustion compounded everything.

A year before, I had started a walking/exercise routine in order to lose weight. Even though I tried to keep it going during the first few months my husband was away, the added pressures and responsibilities started to eat up my walking time.

But I knew I needed it. So I got back out there in the early mornings when everyone was asleep, despite my lack of sleep. The fresh air, exercise, and time for me were just what I needed. I refocused and was able to manage things better.

Just when we got ourselves into a routine, we had a hiccup.

It was the end of summer, five months into my husband's job situation. While riding his bike, my younger son fell and broke his leg. And it wasn't just a "simple" break. It was a break that required a three-night stay in the hospital, surgery, multiple casts—the works—to eventually come home with a cast from his groin to his toes.

No fun for an eight-year-old kid entering grade three.

Once he was home and settled, with help from my sister, my other son—the saint—and my husband on weekends, we got ourselves into a new routine. Hoisting wheelchairs and walkers, learning crutches, figuring out stairs and bathing were challenges we mastered together.

Crawling into bed exhausted, the silence of the night weighed down on me, fuelling my ever-racing thoughts. When I would finally get to sleep after an hour or two of worrying about everyone and everything, I would wake up only a few short hours later. My morning exercise routine dwindled away again.

I had my boys to worry about; I wasn't the important one here. Trying to maintain happiness and balance while navigating this new way of living was most important.

Within a month, we were once again on track, and I resumed my desperately needed early morning walks. And this time, I had a plan for tackling my stress.

When I went to bed, I would visualize the path I would take the next morning, seeing every tree, house and landmark along the way. Doing so relaxed me, driving away worries that raced around my mind. Yes, I had days and nights when I still felt overwhelmed and my sleep was broken. But I kept walking, telling myself that things weren't really that bad, remembering this was only temporary. This too would pass. It could have been so much worse, and I was fortunate with what I did have. Heck, if my son could endure a broken leg and surgeries, I could handle this. My self-talk and visualization worked and, combined with my walks, I started to feel better as our routine and life levelled out.

September, October, then November flew by. Then winter hit—big.

Severe ice, snow and cold temperatures brought our city, unused to harsh winters, to a standstill. My older son and I shovelled snow while my younger son, now with a different cast, watched from the confines of a sled. Getting the boys to and from school, never mind me to work, was a challenge. Trying to navigate a casted boy over icy sidewalks and parking lots was no easy feat. And of course my walks were non-existent.

Then the car broke down.

Just keep it coming, I thought.

Not once, not twice, but three times the tow truck saved me in the harsh, icy conditions. I might as well have had a reserved spot at the repair shop. With being snowed in, worrying about the car, and my poor kid stuck with a cast, I did the best I could to keep my spirits up. But I started heading back to that stressed-out fog.

The snow melted, as snow, too, is only temporary, and the car was eventually fixed.

December left us, leading us to January and milder temperatures. I was determined to get back to my walking routine, and I did. Another operation on my son's leg in February, then the cast was off. The car still ran, and my other son, the saint, seemed no worse for wear.

Anything else was manageable.

I kept walking. With every step, I pounded out whatever current situation was bothering me. Sometimes forcing myself, when my bed was too comfy or I felt too tired, to get out there and clear my head. I realized while I needed to take care of everyone else, if I was going to cope with whatever came my way, I had to take care of myself as well. My boys had fared well through those times, their resilience and independence, and mine, tested and strengthened.

With each step, the proverbial "one step at a time" came to mind.

If I could manage what I had in the previous months, I could do anything—we could do anything. Letting stress deprive me of sleep and interfere with my sanity only gave it power. I was stronger than that, and I got stronger with every step.

— Lisa McManus Lange —

Me and Lady Gaga

Stress and I have been best friends for a long time. As a result of befriending stress, I have had three wrecks, chronic pain, high blood pressure and headaches that paralyze me. My job as a hospice chaplain is hard, stressful and offers me little time to relax and care for myself.

I knew when I lay flat on my back in the hospital parking lot with three broken bones in my left ankle, something had to change.

I re-evaluated my work, my life goals, my schedule and my lack of self-care. I created a schedule that allowed me to have more time at home, more time to exercise and I began eating healthier.

Those were all good changes to combat stress. But the gift my daughters gave me was the best tool of all.

I am not a technology gadget kind of person and the Beatles were my favorite musical group growing up. So when I unwrapped the gift of an iPod full of music my girls selected for their fifty-something-year-old mother, I was surprised.

They explained that this gift of an iPod was to help me use music to calm myself down, energize me when working out, and keep me on an upbeat path. It took me a while to learn how to use it, but once I did, I was hooked!

Of all the songs they put on it, I somehow have gravitated to the music of Lady Gaga. I can't figure out how this middle-aged, somewhat conservative woman from the South has found Lady Gaga's sound so welcoming and invigorating. Yes, I don't understand all the words, but when I hear "Bad Romance" come on, I step a bit faster on the treadmill. "Poker Face" makes me smile and "Born This Way" just makes me want to dance!

Music is certainly a tool for coping with stress and the little iPod I carry with me every day is a constant reminder of the love my girls have for me and my need to take time to tap my feet, clap my hands, roll my head and dance along this road of life. Music is a small thing that makes a big difference in my life. And while I may not wear meat as a dress, or balloons as a cover, I certainly do like the way I feel listening to Lady Gaga's music. It transforms me from the reality of my world and allows me to escape just long enough to rid myself of toxic thoughts and feelings of stress.

I don't understand why it works; I just understand that it does.

— Malinda Dunlap Fillingim —

The Ladies
of the Gym

After my retirement, I was edgy, tired and was developing a few aches and pains—probably arthritis, because, after all, I was old. I was retired, wasn't I? I knew I was stressed, but unaware of a new kind of stress insidiously revealing itself when I stopped working. I was no longer trying to balance children, career and all the usual worries and irritants (joys too, of course) involved: too much work, too many people, too many demands, and so on. That was my old life. Although annoying and aggravating, hassles such as those were not the only villains that produce stress.

It was too quiet. It was too peaceful and I was... yes... bored. I found myself wandering around the house, worrying about all the chores that I could and should be doing now that I had "the time," but invariably put off because, well, there was no hurry, no deadline, no emergency. Apathy had set in big-time. I realized that although most people associate hyperactivity and agitation with stress, my present state of lethargy was a big, red flag. I came to the conclusion that I was suffering from this new (to me) kind of stress. It was invading my life and I'd better deal with it.

We all know the many ways that are recommended for dealing with stress: deep breathing, yoga, a nice, long, restful vacation, doing good deeds for others, and exercise. I chose exercise. I was trying not to listen to what my brain was telling me—something like, "You? Work out? Hah!" True, I do not enjoy that ritual, the phenomenon that has overtaken so many in recent years, called "going to the gym." Being an RN, I know how vital exercise is for our overall health and wellbeing, but something about relying on machines to tone us, slim us, and awaken those endorphins in our overburdened brains simply wasn't my thing. I liked the natural approach, such as a simple daily walk, dancing or washing windows. But I was not doing any of those things and knew I was in trouble. Drastic measures were called for! Hence the gym. And what happened there surprised even me, old and seasoned as I was.

The first day at the gym, which catered to women, I received the usual instructions, then silently but unhappily put in my half hour and went home. The second day I looked around and noticed a few women who had been there the day before. The third day I hesitantly began to speak, commenting on the weather and other such bland subjects. Day after day the same women were there and I began to think of them as "the ladies of the gym."

One day somebody commented on a shocking event in the news that morning. Suddenly we were all talking at once, sharing our opinions, some a little more cautiously than others. But as time went on, we all became fearless in speaking about almost everything.

I began to look forward to sharing the day's news with "the ladies." It became apparent that after our workouts—during which we vented, sometimes vehemently, sometimes more delicately—I began to feel more relaxed. The tension in my shoulders lessened, and my constant fatigue had all but disappeared. True, exercise can and does have this effect. But my eagerness to get to the gym had very little to do with the workout and had very much to do with the anticipation of discussing the news and the camaraderie that ensued.

My funny, outspoken, irascible ladies! At first, they were just the ladies at the gym. Now they are my personal antidote for stress. They put a smile on my face and a spring in my step. They make me laugh. They make me think. They make me care. They make me come to the gym each day and love it! The ladies of the gym are now my friends.

As I write this, it is early morning. I am sitting at my kitchen table with a cup of coffee, relaxed and almost stress-free, eagerly planning the things I will accomplish this day and of course gathering up juicy tidbits from the TV news to discuss... no... to rant and rave about later today with the ladies of the gym.

~ Catherine Ring Saliba ~

De-stress
Your Lifestyle

Introduction

In times of stress the resolve to live a healthy lifestyle is often one of the first things to fall by the wayside. I mean, have you ever tried to stick to a sensible diet when you're under an intense deadline or after an upsetting spat with a co-worker? Most people don't reach for a carrot to calm jitters in these kinds of situations.

Actually, overeating is a perfect example of how stress breeds some of the worst lifestyle behavior. A lot of emotional eaters use food as a form of self-medication, literally soothing feelings of anger, depression, anxiety and sadness with too much food. On a chemical level, stress increases output of the hormone cortisol, which stimulates cravings for fatty, sweet and salty "comfort" foods. And for some, stress eating has been their go-to coping mechanism since childhood and might even be considered a family tradition.

Other weak moments tend to follow similar patterns for similar reasons. Anyone with an undesirable health habit will be the first to admit that stress and vice seem to go hand in hand — and round and round. One of the most common reactions to a highly stressful episode is indulgence in the wrong things. This weakens the mind and body in a myriad of ways that open the door to additional stress and in turn, ups the urge to overindulge again. It's a vicious cycle that can be hard to break.

I definitely think it's worth taking a look at your lifestyle practices as part of any serious stress reduction effort. Healthier living is one of the simplest and least expensive ways to cope with stress and counteract its negative effects. In fact, it's essential. I think all of the storytellers in this chapter would agree! So let's review some basic changes that can make a significant difference in how you respond to life's pressures.

Clean Up Your Act

Obviously food isn't the only way people self-medicate. Smoking, excessive drinking, drugs and self-harming behaviors are other common less-than-healthy coping mechanisms. Self-medication is an attempt to relieve problems such as anxiety, pain, sleeplessness or perhaps the symptoms of something bigger such as clinical depression or post-traumatic stress disorder. The benefits of self-medicating are usually short lived while the additional problems it stirs up are potentially long-term and highly destructive.

Are you concerned that your self-medicating may be getting out of hand? If so, ask yourself the following questions: Has anyone ever questioned your self-medication? If you told your doctor about your self-medicating behavior, would she question it? Does your habit of self-medicating cost you more money than it does ten other people you know? Do you need more of the substance or activity each time to get the soothing benefit? Is self-medication disruptive to your relationships, work or other major aspects of your life? If you answer yes to any of these questions, I recommend you speak to a professional to help you get your behavior—and stress—under control.

Don't Worry. Be Happy.

Just as stress weakens the resolve to be healthy, it can also sap your ability to enjoy life. Busy, stressed out people report having less time for their families, hobbies, sex with their partners—or really, any fun at all. That's a shame because there's a scientific notion that doing something pleasurable can do more than just bring you pleasure.

A brand new area of research shows how enjoyment reduces stress by inhibiting the brain's anxiety response. Catherine Ring Saliba with her ladies at the gym and Malinda Fillingim with her Lady Gaga are good examples of how this works. As for the research to back this up, when University of Cincinnati researchers fed rats tasty foods or gave them free access to the opposite sex they had lower levels of stress hormones and slower heart rates than rats that weren't allowed to live the high life. The happiness benefits lasted for seven days.

True, humans aren't rats. But the researchers believe the same rules apply to people. Taking some time to do something for the sheer joy of it can turn out to be a pretty effective way to blow off some steam. Even the simple act of getting in a good belly laugh on a regular basis has been shown to significantly decrease stress hormones.

I realize that in this productivity-driven, multitasking world of ours it's hard not to feel a twinge of guilt when you stop for 15 minutes to read a book or take a walk "just because." Do what Lisa McManus Lange eventually did — ditch the guilt and do it anyway. Having a hobby, a passion or even just time for yourself will allow you to decompress and tune into something other than your problems.

Sleep It Off

If you lie awake at night tossing and turning, replaying negative thoughts over and over, stress is definitely taking a toll on your health. An occasional sleepless night or one extra-long nap probably won't do you in but it won't do you any favors either. A recent University of Pennsylvania study found that subjects who slept only 4.5 hours for one week reported feeling more stressed, angry, sad, and mentally exhausted. When the subjects resumed normal sleep, their moods improved. Numerous other studies reveal that persistent sleep problems hamper your ability to deal with stress as well as affect problem solving, memory and a host of other cognitive functions.

On the flip side, feeling agitated isn't conducive to sleep. Stress often translates into being aroused, awake, and alert, which is why people who are under constant stress or who have abnormally exaggerated responses to stress tend to have sleep problems. Difficulty with sleep is often the first sign of depression or some other mental issue.

Experts aren't sure what the magic sleep number is for health and stress reduction. Research indicates that it's probably somewhere between seven and nine hours of uninterrupted sleep per night but what's optimal can vary widely for each individual. If you frequently feel groggy and unrefreshed and feel this hampers your ability to manage stress, it's worth addressing your problems with sleep.

Sweating Off Stress

You may recall that in Chapter 6, I explained how stress activates the sympathetic nervous system's flight-or-fight response to elevate heart rate, spike blood pressure and increase blood flow. Our ancestors depended on this reaction to flee the physical dangers they faced on a daily basis but in today's world this reaction usually has nowhere to go, so instead it churns through the mind and body wreaking physical and mental havoc.

Exercise is one of the few ways we have of clearing the chemical byproducts of stress from the body. In essence, it provides the opportunity for flight — or if you practice a discipline like martial arts, fight — and this helps restore the body's systems to their pre-stress state. Some experts also believe that exercise promotes the release of endorphins, the so-called happy hormones that elicit tranquil feelings; however, current research has shown this effect may not be as powerful as was once thought after the first few weeks of regular activity. One new theory that deserves further attention is that the positive stress of exercise prepares cells, structures and pathways within the brain so that they're more equipped to handle stress in other forms.

It really doesn't matter why exercise beats stress since it's crystal clear that it does. Studies correlating stress levels to health status find that fitter people are more capable of managing stress than people who don't move on a regular basis. And in surveys gym rats usually report lower levels of stress than couch dwellers. Many people experience immediate mood improvements after a single, moderately paced bout of exercise. More lasting stress reduction benefits appear to kick in after just a few weeks. A consistent exercise routine is probably what helped Rachel Moore adjust to being the family's breadwinner.

The research indicates that cardiovascular exercise like walking, jogging and swimming works best for calming the nerves, but I suspect this is because it's the type of exercise most often examined in studies. As scientists turn their attention to the stress-busting benefits of stretching, strength training and stop-and-go activities like tennis, I think the evidence will mount in their favor too. Most experts recommend doing 30 minutes of moderate intensity physical activity you enjoy as many days of the week as possible.

Edible Stress Busters

Though there's some solid evidence certain foods help neutralize stress, I'm a little skeptical of stress busting diet plans. There's no proof that putting specific foods together in a specific combination will magically melt away negative emotions and thoughts, any more than they will melt away pounds. That said, I do believe it makes sense to load up your diet with foods that give you a fighting chance of fighting stress—and living a healthy life.

Different foods help counteract stress in different ways. Some reduce stress by raising the level of feel-good hormones that help you feel calm while others lower the levels of stress hormones that rattle your nerves. Others contain natural sedatives such as tryptophan or nutrients that enhance your autoimmune response, counteract cell damage or reduce blood pressure. Some good examples of edible stress relievers: Foods high in vitamin C such as blueberries, oranges, and leafy green vegetables have been shown to help reduce tension. Studies indicate that fish, walnuts and other foods rich in omega-3 fatty acids may help fight depression. Peaches, poultry and dairy all contain different types of natural sedatives that may help reduce anxiety. Also, anything that's high in fiber (fruits, veggies, nuts, whole grains) can help regulate blood sugar to prevent mood swings. In general anything that's good for your body in others ways will help combat stress.

Many foods can help mellow you out but not all of them in a healthy way. Simple carbohydrates, fats and super salty treats may serve as comfort foods in the moment; however, they can lead to weight gain and poor health sapping your defenses to deal with stress in the future. Studies provide a strong hint that the magnesium and other substances found in chocolate keep you happy but too much of a good thing will dump an excess of fat, sugar and calories into your diet. (Dark chocolate is the best choice since it's lower in fat, sugar and calories than other chocolates and also boasts the highest levels of feel-good chemicals.)

Chicken Soup for the Stressed-Out Soul

Grandma was right when she told you there is nothing more soothing than chicken soup. Now she has the science to back up her words! In a recent experiment, University of Buffalo researchers discovered that feeding someone a steaming bowl of chicken soup helped decrease feelings of loneliness and reminded people about close relationships. I love this research and I'd like to suggest chicken soup can nourish your stressed-out soul in many ways.

I've created a recipe here for you (with the help of my friends at Dietsinreview.com) chock full of antioxidants, vitamin C and other stress-busting nutrients. Why not cook a pot for yourself—or better yet, to share with your loved ones—on a regular basis?

Think about how relaxing it is to stroll down the aisles of a supermarket or farmers market, selecting these wonderful, health-giving ingredients. Picture lovingly chopping, dicing and preparing the recipe. Imagine the delightful smell filling your home as the soup simmers on the stove. Now, dress your table in its finest tablecloth, china and silverware. Add a fresh loaf of bread from your local bakery. Then sit down and share the goodness of your creation with the people you love. Has there ever been a more beautiful ritual for easing stress and reaffirming all that it is important in your life?

Chicken Noodle
and Sweet Potato Soup

This chicken noodle and sweet potato soup is a stress-busting powerhouse. It's loaded with veggies rich in antioxidants and fiber to keep you feeling your best all the time.

Serves 6
Serving Size: 2 cups

Ingredients:
16 oz low-sodium chicken broth
1/2 chicken bouillon cube
1 cup sweet onion, chopped (contains flavanoids,
    polyphenols, chromium, vitamin C, and fiber)
1 1/2 cups celery, chopped (contains vitamin K, vitamin C,
    potassium, folate, fiber, and molybdenum)
1 1/2 cup carrots, chopped (contains carotenoids, poly-
    acetylenes, vitamin C, and fiber)
1/2 pound chicken breast, cooked and diced (contains
    protein, niacin, selenium, vitamin B6, and phosphorus)
6 oz egg noodles
1 medium sweet potato, diced (contains vitamin A, vitamin
    C, and fiber)
1 tsp garlic, minced (contains manganese, vitamin B, and
    vitamin C)
2 tbsp extra virgin olive oil

I tsp rosemary, fresh (contains compounds that have been linked to increasing blood flow to the brain, improving concentration)

I tsp thyme, fresh (contains vitamin K and iron; considered to have healing effects because of carvacolo, borneol, geraniol, and thymol compounds)

Pepper, to taste

Directions:

1. Heat the extra virgin olive oil in a stockpot.
2. Add the onion, celery, and carrots to the pot. Sauté for approximately 2 minutes or until onions become translucent.
3. Add the chicken broth, bouillon cube, garlic, rosemary, and thyme to the pot. Bring ingredients to a steady boil.
4. Add the chicken breast and the noodles to the pot. Cover and let simmer on medium-high heat for 20 minutes. Stir occasionally.
5. Sprinkle with pepper.
6. Serve and enjoy!

Nutrition Information:

Calories: 140.5 kcals; Total Fat: 6 grams; Saturated Fat: 1 grams; Carbohydrates: 17.7 grams; Fiber: 2.4 grams; protein: 5.1 grams; cholesterol: 11.9 milligrams; sodium: 165 milligram.

(49% Carb, 14% Protein. 37% Fat)

Meet Our Contributors

Beth Arvin began writing plays for her siblings and neighborhood friends in grammar school. Currently she writes a daily blog, betharvin365.livejournal.com, and a blog, "I Think So," for the *Kent Reporter*. She is hoping to complete her first novel by mid 2012. E-mail her at betharvin@gmail.com.

John P. Buentello writes essays, fiction, and poetry. He is the coauthor of the novel *Reproduction Rights* and the short story collection *Binary Tales*. Currently he is at work on a new novel. E-mail him at jakkhakk@yahoo.com.

Dianne E. Butts has over 275 publications in magazines and books. She is the author of *Deliver Me* and *Dear America* and is an aspiring screenwriter. Dianne enjoys riding her motorcycle with her husband Hal and gardening with her cat P.C. in Colorado. Learn more at www.DianneEButts.com and www.DeliverMeBook.com.

Jane McBride Choate has been weaving stories in her head for as long as she can remember. Being in the *Chicken Soup for the Soul* series is a dream come true for her.

Harriet Cooper is a freelance writer. Her topics often include health, exercise, diet, cats, family and the environment. A frequent contributor to the *Chicken Soup for the Soul* series, her work has also appeared in newspapers, magazines, newsletters, anthologies, websites and on the radio. Contact her via e-mail at shewrites@ live.ca.

Priscilla Dann-Courtney is a writer and clinical psychologist living in Boulder with her husband and three children. She recently published her first book, *Room to Grow: Stories of Life and Family*, which is a collection of her essays. Her passions include family, friends, writing, yoga, running and baking.

Malinda Dunlap Fillingim is now listening to her iPod in Leland, NC, where she continues to dance and sing while looking for a job—a very stressful experience! E-mail her at fillingam@ ec.rr.com.

Dana Hill is a freelance writer, professional bartender, and passionate cook living in Oakland, CA. Her work has appeared in *Chicken Soup for the Soul* books and in travel anthologies published by the writing collective Townsend 11 (townsend11. com). Dana holds a Bachelor of Arts degree in architecture from UC Berkeley.

Mary Hughes loves to write true stories that bring laughter to the heart and inspiration to the soul. She is also a devotional writer. Her newsletter, *Christian Potpourri*, is in its ninth year.

After a thirty-five-year marriage, creating a nonprofit charity, and coping with her son's lung cancer as well as her own chronic illness, **Marsha Jordan** is no stranger to difficulties. She shares some hard-earned wisdom, along with a few laughs, in her book, *Hugs, Hope, and Peanut Butter.* Contact her via e-mail at jordans@newnorth.net.

April Knight is proud to be a contributor to the *Chicken Soup for the Soul* series. She is currently writing romance novels for people over fifty. April spends her days riding horses and her nights writing mystery novels. She also writes a newspaper column and novels under her tribal name Crying Wind Hummingbird.

Jeannie Lancaster, a freelance writer from Loveland, CO, recognizes the restorative power nature has when one is dealing with stress. She finds quiet moments spent among God's creations a healing peace and gentle inspiration for much of her writing.

Lisa McManus Lange walks regularly to pound out the stress — and to mastermind what to write next. The cast sits in the closet. A previous *Chicken Soup for the Soul* contributor, she lives with her family in Victoria, BC, Canada. E-mail her at lisamc2010@yahoo.ca or visit her at www.lisamcmanuslange. blogspot.com.

Eve Legato is a graduate of Hampshire College. She has since worked for a theatre company, a law firm, and a publishing house. Her beagle, Zeus, is her favorite stress reliever.

Teena Maenza is an award-winning journalist and freelance writer living in West Columbia, TX. Her husband, children and grandchildren have always been her greatest sources of inspiration.

John McCutcheon retired after many years in health administration, some as Superintendent in a mission hospital. He currently works part-time as a doctor in an AIDS clinic and delights to see patients recovering. He enjoys writing a column for a local newspaper and other creative challenges. E-mail him at j.mcc@webmail.co.za.

Marie-Therese Miller and her husband, John, are the proud parents of five. She is the author of nonfiction books for children and teenagers, including the *Dog Tales* series, *Managing Responsibilities*, and *Rachel Carson*. Her stories have appeared in several *Chicken Soup for the Soul* volumes. Learn more at www.marie-theresemiller.com.

Nina Schatzkamer Miller lives in Olivette, MO, with her husband and three sons. She enjoyed her work as the Children's Area Specialist at Borders and is now doing story time at her local community center and writing a handbook to help others with their story times. Contact her at www.ultimatestorytime.com.

Rachel L. Moore has a BSEE degree, but wears many hats. She is a wife, mother, an engineer, inventor, writer, author, dancer, speaker, and life coach. Rachel enjoys providing success tools and training to help individuals, families, entrepreneurs, educators, and organizations transform desires and goals into reality. Contact her at www.mindyourvision.com.

Shirley Dunn Perry is a nurse and author of *Ten Five-Minute Miracles: How to Relax*. Her work has appeared in many publications. Biscuit making, hiking, world travel, watercolors, and enjoying her family and grandchildren add zest to her writing adventures. E-mail her at sdunnperry@gmail.com. Blog: shirleydunnperry.wordpress.com.

Connie Pombo is an inspirational author, speaker and freelance writer. She has contributed several stories to the *Chicken Soup for the Soul* series and is the author of *Living and Retiring in Cuenca: 101 Questions Answered*. Connie and her husband, Mark, now call Cuenca, Ecuador home. Contact her at www.conniepombo.com.

Catherine Ring Saliba is a University of Vermont graduate, retired R.N., proud grandmother, and TV and film actress. She now joyfully pursues writing, and her work has been published in several magazines and newspapers. This is her second story in the *Chicken Soup for the Soul* series. E-mail her at ringsal@aol.com.

Sarah Jo Smith holds a master's degree in education. She has taught high school English and instructed adult literature classes. She writes short stories and essays and is currently seeking an agent for her first novel, *Well Kept Secrets*, while working on her second novel. She lives in Bend, OR, with her husband.

Marilyn Turk received her B.A. degree in journalism from LSU and has been published in *Guideposts*, *The Upper Room*, *Clubhouse Jr.*, *Coastal Christian Family*, and *Chicken Soup for the Soul* books. She and husband Chuck enjoy fishing and playing tennis. She is writing a Christian historical novel. Learn more at Pathwayheart.com.

Judy A. Weist is a writer who uses her experiences of everyday life to fill the pages of her short stories and memoirs. She delights in teaching dance to young children and loves to write. Her story "No Place Like Home" appeared in *Chicken Soup: Inspiration for the Young at Heart*. Contact her via e-mail at weistjudy@yahoo.com.

Meet Our Authors

Dr. Jeff Brown is an Instructor in the Department of Psychiatry at Harvard Medical School where he's been on faculty for over a decade. Dr. Brown is a Clinical Associate at McLean Hospital, the largest psychiatric affiliate of Harvard Medical School. He is board certified by the American Board of Professional Psychology in both Clinical Psychology and Cognitive & Behavioral Psychology. Additionally, he is a member of the United States Olympic Committee's Registry of Psychologists, is the medical team psychologist for the Boston Marathon, and serves on *Runner's World* magazine's scientific advisory board. In 2010, Dr. Brown received an honorary doctorate from the University of Central Missouri for his professional contributions to psychology and science.

Dr. Brown is the author or coauthor of two books including the bestselling title *The Winner's Brain: 8 Strategies Great Minds Use to Achieve Success* (DaCapo, 2010) and *The Competitive Edge: How to Win Every Time You Compete* (Tyndale, 2007). His next book, *Chicken Soup for the Soul: Think Positive for Great Health*, will be published in September 2012. He has also authored academic book chapters and journal articles. His witty and indispensable messages are frequently heard by audiences at conferences and events across the globe. When he's not writing or seeing clients in his office, you will find him working out at the gym, fishing or biking, or enjoying breakfast with his family at their neighborhood diner. Visit his interactive website for timely and practical resources at www.DrJeffBrown.com.

Liz Neporent is a health, fitness and medical writer who has written more than 15 books including the bestsellers *The Winner's Brain: 8 Strategies Great Minds Use to Achieve Success* and *Weight Training for Dummies*. She is a regular contributor to dozens of websites, publications and national media outlets. She is on the emeritus board of directors and a national spokesperson for the American Council on Exercise and the fitness and social media advisor for The Hudson Valley Women's Health Initiative, a charitable organization dedicated to educating people about medical, health and fitness. She lives in New York City with her husband Jay and daughter Skylar. Follow her on twitter @lizzyfit or check out her website www.liznep.com.

Acknowledgments

Walden Pond, surrounded by a patch of woods not far from Boston, is famously known because of Henry David Thoreau. Thoreau lived in a slight, hand-forged cabin just off the northwestern banks of the pond from 1845 to 1847 because he "...*wished to live deliberately, to front only the essential facts of life...*" So, he shaped his lifestyle from nature, and eventually wrote prolifically about it. I suppose you could say Thoreau went head to head with stress just to see what would happen, hoping he'd understand himself and life a little bit better as a result.

Like Thoreau's important quest, the writing and production of *Say Goodbye to Stress* wasn't always stress-free either. The book you're getting to read is a product of stress management — and fun. Perhaps Thoreau was braver than me going it alone in the forest. Rather, I had tremendous support and resources that I'd like you to know about.

First, as you turn the pages you'll quickly appreciate the writing expertise of Liz Neporent. When you chuckle as you read, you are experiencing Liz's genuine humor. She's a pro at getting in your head. Next, my colleagues at Harvard Health Publications, Drs. Julie Silver and Anthony Komaroff, frequently give me opportunities to try to make differences in people's lives through writing. I'm humbled to support Harvard Health Publications' slogan, "trusted advice for a healthier life." Among other trusted names you know is Chicken Soup for the Soul. My Chicken Soup editor, Amy Newmark, has expertly led a lineup of talented individuals who've thoughtfully shaped every aspect of the book you hold. In addition, she has pored over thousands of significant stories provided by contributing writers in order to capture personal experiences that make the text come alive for you. And on the home front, my wife Carolynne knows and supports every moment I invest in writing. And, I love her for giving me that freedom.

Chicken Soup for the Soul and Harvard Medical School have a strong, unique collaboration that you can rely on. Undoubtedly, we want your life to be improved. Along the way, you can bet we've passed around jokes about the irony of being stressed while publishing a book about stress. Our jokes never seem to get old. What also stays fresh are the powerful insights, clever strategies, and personal victories which have come from going head to head with stress on your behalf. Like Thoreau, we set out to learn about life, then write about it. Thoreau once said, *"Everyone must believe in something. I believe I'll go canoeing."* Now that's a great way to Say Goodbye to Stress.

Say Goodbye to Stress is dedicated to Marie Hill, a dear family friend who holds fast to a worry-free faith and has given immeasurably to others for nearly a century. She has been nurse, neighbor, problem-solver and *Granny* to many.

More Great Stories and
Medical Advice from

Chicken Soup
for the Soul ®

and doctors at

HARVARD
MEDICAL
SCHOOL

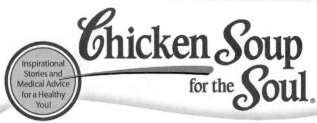

Inspirational Stories and Medical Advice for a Healthy You!

Chicken Soup
for the Soul.

by **DR. JEFF BROWN** of
HARVARD MEDICAL SCHOOL

Think Positive
for
Great
Health

Use Your Mind to Promote Your Own Healing and Wellness

Solid advice and transformative stories —
a true path to a positive outlook and great health!
~ Dr. Arthur J. Siegel

Chicken Soup for the Soul:
Think Positive for Great Health
978-1-935096-90-0
ebook: 978-1-611592-13-9

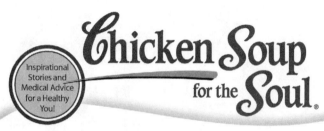

Chicken Soup for the Soul

for the Soul.

Inspirational Stories and Medical Advice for a Healthy You!

by DR. MARIE PASINSKI of HARVARD MEDICAL SCHOOL
with LIZ NEPORENT

Boost Your Brain Power!

You Can Improve and Energize Your Brain at Any Age

*A great guide to powering up your brain...
and I loved the motivational stories too!*
~ Dr. Joe Shrand

*Chicken Soup for the Soul:
Boost Your Brain Power!*
978-1-935096-86-3
ebook: 978-1-611592-10-8

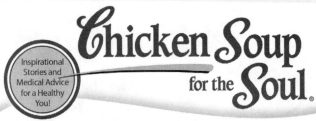

by DR. JULIE SILVER of HARVARD MEDICAL SCHOOL

Say Goodbye to Back Pain!

How to Handle Flare-Ups, Injuries, and Everyday Back Health

Terrific tips for flare-ups and for chronic back pain. You'll be back in action sooner than you think!
~ Dr. Howard Ezra Lewine

Chicken Soup for the Soul:
Say Goodbye to Back Pain!
978-1-935096-87-0
ebook: 978-1-611592-08-5

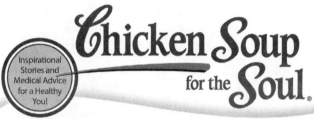
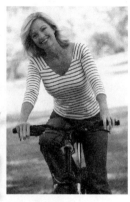

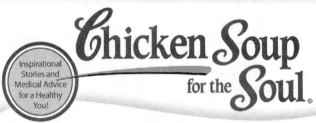

Chicken Soup for the Soul®

Inspirational Stories and Medical Advice for a Healthy You!

by **DR. JULIE SILVER** of
HARVARD MEDICAL SCHOOL

Hope & Healing
for Your
Breast
Cancer
Journey

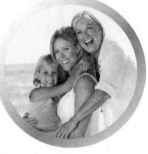

Surviving and Thriving During and After
Your Diagnosis and Treatment

Every woman diagnosed with breast cancer
deserves excellent emotional and medical support—
this book delivers both! ~Dr. Kimberly Allison

Chicken Soup for the Soul:
Hope & Healing for Your Breast Cancer Journey
978-1-935096-94-8
ebook: 978-1-611592-11-5